HERBAL ANTIVIRALS

Heal Yourself Faster, Cheaper and Safer

Your A-Z Guide to Choosing, Preparing and Using the Most Effective Natural Antiviral Herbs

By Mary Jones

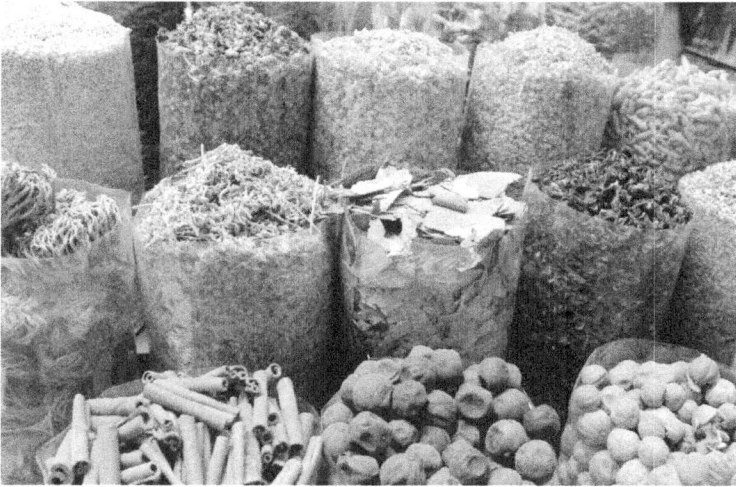

"The healing comes from nature and not from the physician. Therefore the physician Must start from nature with an open mind"

- Paracelsus

TABLE OF CONTENTS

INTRODUCTION

Are you feeling overwhelmed by constant viral infections? Struggling to get your head around the concept of alternative remedies – and particularly herbs – as restorative antivirals?

Or do you want to fully understand the role of *herbalism* in an age where there's always another emerging killer virus – think coronavirus, MERS, Ebola, etc. – and fully protect yourself?

If so, you're in the right place.

You see, plants have been used as the basis of medication throughout human history to **help prevent and cure a wide range of ailments**. These remedies are recognized in modern medicine as '*alternative treatments*' and have been steadily increasing in popularity for many reasons. One of the reasons, according to the *Journal of Traditional and Complementary Medicine*, is the simple fact that there are no preventive vaccines or efficient antiviral therapies to control these ailments. Also, the fact that viruses tend to mutate fast and become more dangerous (something that may render existing vaccines ineffective) makes it worse.

Scary revelation, huh?

According to the *Journal*, *"Identifying novel antiviral drugs is of critical importance and natural products are an excellent source for such discoveries."*

That simply means that although antiviral medication is important, it isn't always the answer. To prevent a growing resistance to the work of prescription medication, **herbal remedies are brilliant for prevention – and cure** when the virus isn't life-threatening. Research has actually proven this – for instance, I'm sure you've heard of antivirals like:

- Oregano oil, which has been used for ages to reduce the activity of stomach flu through its potent carvacrol compounds.
- Basil, which has been used to fight herpes viruses, enterovirus, and hepatitis B courtesy of ursolic acid, apigenin, and other strong compounds.

- Fennel, which, through a powerful component known as trans-anothole, has been used to reduce inflammation, increase immunity, and fight against herpes viruses.

And so many more which are <u>well studied</u> and published in *PubMed Central* (from the *National Institutes of Health*), and <u>proven</u> to fight different kinds of viruses. Beyond that, **herbal remedies are also brilliant for assisting with the side effects of medication**, and it's because of this awareness, empirical data, and all the positive facts that this guide is here.

So if you've been asking questions like:

— *What is the impact of herbal remedies on viruses, including the most recent one (Covid-19), in preventing and treating them?*

— *How has herbalism worked in annihilating viruses in the recent years?*

— *What herbal antivirals are we talking about?*

— *What common ailments are best treated with herbal remedies?*

You'll find all the answers to these and more that might pop up later in this book.

You'll also:

- Get deep insight into the *top herbal antivirals* today, a breakdown and full details of many more that are easily accessible to you.

- Learn the benefits and risks of these remedies.

- Get extensive coverage of the recent, and emerging, viruses (including coronavirus), complete with statistics and refined facts you need to know about them.

And, of course, everything else there is to know about herbal remedies that you'll not find in any other guide.

Once you have read all of the information in the following chapters, **you will be able to make an extremely informed decision about switching to the healthier, more natural alternative of herbal medication!**

Remember, however, that everything presented in this book is only a guideline — you will need to consult your doctor before taking any of these herbal remedies.

Ready to get started?

CHAPTER 1
KEY FACTS ABOUT EMERGING VIRUSES

Every year, more than 2 million people are affected by infections. In the U.S. alone, over 100,000 people die because of infections they acquired in hospitals and health clinics. Some of these can be classified as emergent viruses, which is a viral strain that is newly discovered or one that generates a new disease or infection. Most of these can be categorized as '*zoonotic*,' which is when a disease can be transferred from animals to humans.

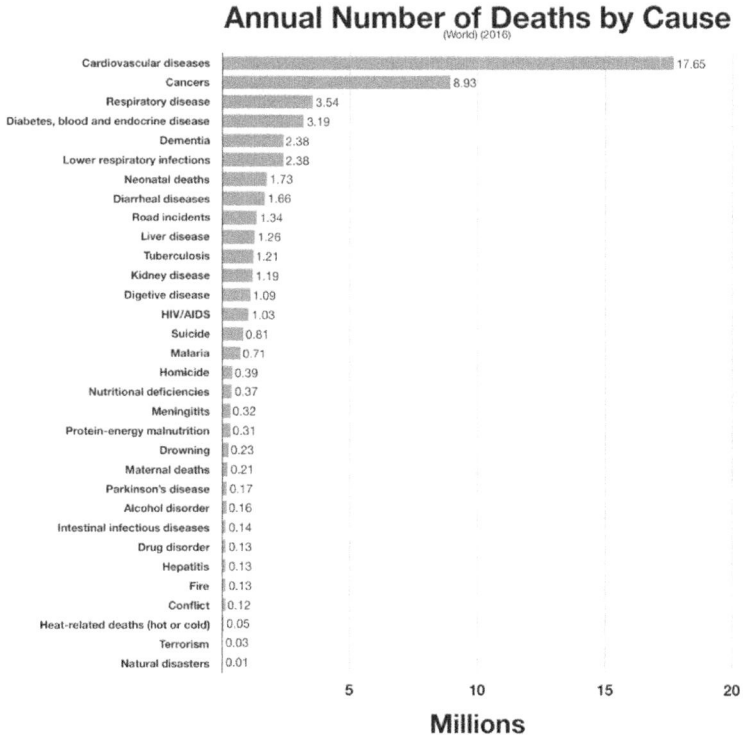

Annual Number of Deaths by Cause
(World) (2016)

Cause	Millions
Cardiovascular diseases	17.65
Cancers	8.93
Respiratory disease	3.54
Diabetes, blood and endocrine disease	3.19
Dementia	2.38
Lower respiratory infections	2.38
Neonatal deaths	1.73
Diarrheal diseases	1.66
Road incidents	1.34
Liver disease	1.26
Tuberculosis	1.21
Kidney disease	1.19
Digetive disease	1.09
HIV/AIDS	1.03
Suicide	0.81
Malaria	0.71
Homicide	0.39
Nutritional deficiencies	0.37
Meningitits	0.32
Protein-energy malnutrition	0.31
Drowning	0.23
Maternal deaths	0.21
Parkinson's disease	0.17
Alcohol disorder	0.16
Intestinal infectious diseases	0.14
Drug disorder	0.13
Hepatitis	0.13
Fire	0.13
Conflict	0.12
Heat-related deaths (hot or cold)	0.05
Terrorism	0.03
Natural disasters	0.01

Millions

The *factors that affect emerging viruses* are:

- *Population movements* – the temporary or permanent migration of a specific group of people.
- *Deforestation* – natural forests are cleared through logging or burning.
- *Irrigation* – the artificial application of water to assist the production of crops.
- *Urbanization* – the increase of population in urban areas.
- *Air Travel* – increase in long-distance traveling for both humans and livestock.

A great example of an emerging virus is **Poliomyelitis**. It has been known to exist for centuries without any real impact, but it became more prominent in the 19th century due to dense urban populations forcing people to live so closely together. This wasn't resolved until the vaccine was invented.

Of course, more recent examples of emerging viruses are **AIDS** and **Ebola**. *Dr. Leonard Horowitz* has recently done a very in-depth study on this very topic. Dr. Horowitz received a doctorate in dental medicine from Tufts University alongside master's degrees in behavioral science and health education, from Harvard University and Beacon College respectively. He is often cited as an authority within conversations about behavioral science and public health education. His experience also includes serving as a faculty member at Tufts University, Harvard University, and the Institute for the Arts and Human Development at Leslie College and spending more than a decade directing a multidisciplinary health center. Dr. Horowitz is currently the president of a non-profit corporation focusing on health education.

He starts his study by saying, *"To do evil a human being must first of all believe what he is doing is good...,"* which demonstrates the perspective on human interference in these emerging viruses. His work examines how a lot of these **emerging viruses are not just mutations, but actually man-made**. The implications of this, of course, means that we need to be extremely aware of how we can protect ourselves naturally from this type of thing. If we can incorporate specific foods and herbs into our everyday diet, this gives us a better chance of fighting whatever comes our way.

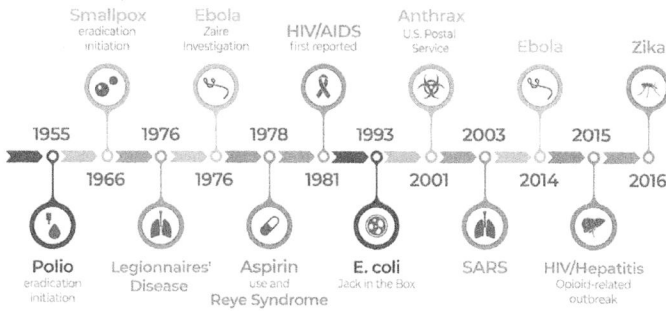

Now that we have had a brief look at the origin of these emerging viruses, it is time to examine what is important – **curing them**. Most people will automatically think of traditional, man-made medication, but this guide will demonstrate how herbal, more natural medication has extensive benefits of its own.

Respiratory Infections – such as the *influenza virus* – are believed to be one of the main reasons that people visit their doctor or pharmacist. According to the NHS (www.nhs.uk), health professionals make the following differentiation:

- *Lower Respiratory Tract Infections* – lungs and airways are affected.

- *Upper Respiratory Tract Infections* – sinuses, throat, and nose are affected.

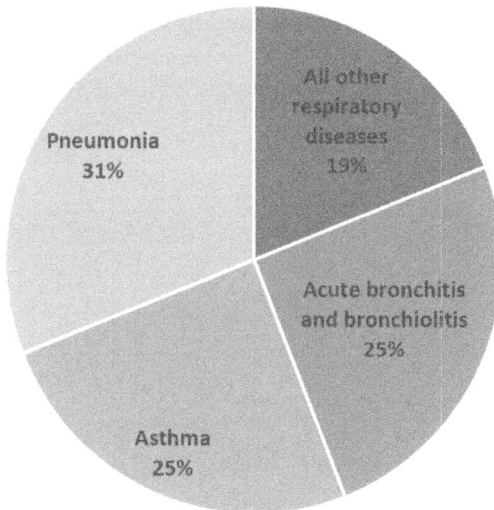

Hospitalizations for Types of Respiratory Diseases, Children Aged less than 15 years, 2005

These viruses can spread in many different ways, most primarily through the air. In fact, droplets carrying the disease are expelled by an infected person whenever they sneeze or cough, and then those droplets can be breathed in by anyone near to them. The only way to attempt to prevent this from happening is by practicing good hygiene.

When suffering an upper respiratory infection, most people chose to treat them at home – which is the best thing to do unless the symptoms continue to worsen or you have underlying health problems. Rest and hydration are key factors in this.

Of course, there are other **medical ways these symptoms can be treated** – or at least alleviated. The most common of these include:

- *Acetaminophen* – (Tylenol) reduces body ache and fever.
- *Nonsteroidal Anti-inflammatory Drugs* – (Ibuprofen) another medication to reduce body ache and fever.
- *Antihistamines* – (Benadryl) can help with nasal congestion.
- *Antitussives* – (Cough Medication) can be used to help with coughing.
- *Steroids* – (Decadron) can be used to reduce inflammation in the airway passage.
- *Decongestants* – (Sudafed) are also good for nasal congestion.
- *Antibiotics* – in some cases, antibiotics will be prescribed.

But there are also many **natural remedies that can help reduce these symptoms**: *Honey, Licorice Root,* and *Thyme* to name a few. These natural solutions will be examined further throughout this guide.

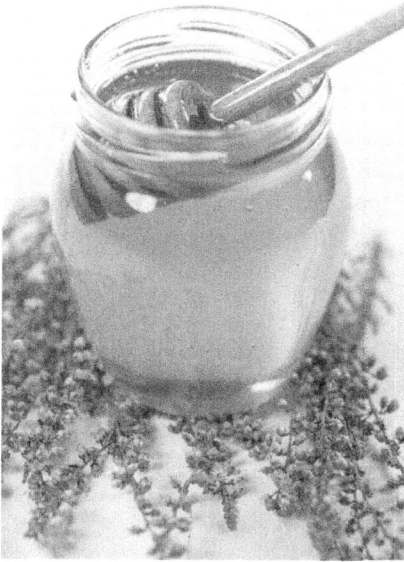

Encephalitis is the medical term defined as inflammation of brain tissue. While a variety of factors could cause this, its most common cause is viral infection (very often it is the herpes simplex virus), but can also be the result of an insect bite. The symptoms of this are usually aching muscles, fever, headaches, fatigue, and nausea – all the common signs that point to a virus. This can often make it very difficult to diagnose, which means victims can slip into a coma. The long-lasting results of this can range from nothing to permanent brain damage. **A few of these issues can include**:

- Problems concentrating.
- Issues with memory.
- Depression, anxiety, and mood imbalance.
- Shifts in personality.
- Behavior issues.
- Persistent headaches.
- Problems swallowing.
- Difficulty speaking.
- Seizures.
- Issues with movement and weakness.
- Difficulty with dexterity, balance, and coordination.

7

Encephalitis has a low rate of occurrence, where approximately 2,500 people are affected annually in Ireland and the UK combined. However, anyone is susceptible, most especially children, the elderly, and people who have had their immune system compromised (for instance, HIV sufferers or people undergoing cancer treatment) are most at risk.

After Encephalitis has been diagnosed using a *Lumbar Puncture* (or spinal tap) or *Electroencephalograph,* which dictates unusual brain waves, then, the antiviral medication **Acyclovir** is traditionally prescribed to assist your body in battling the virus. Doctors will also combine this with 'supportive treatments' such as intravenous fluids to help your body rest and fight.

Although you must be treated by a qualified medical doctor for Encephalitis, there are **natural remedies that you can use to alleviate the symptoms** and strengthen your immune system. These include:

- *Green Tea* – 250-500 mg daily. Being an antioxidant, Green Tea can help boost the immune system and reduce inflammation.
- *Cat's Claw* – 20 mg 3 times per day. Cat's Claw can combat viruses and reduce inflammation.
- *Garlic* – 400 mg 2-3 times a day. Garlic is brilliant for boosting your immune system.
- *Astragalus* – 250-500 mg 4 times a day. Great for boosting your immune system and fighting viruses.
- *Elderberry* – 1-2 spoonfuls of standardized liquid extract 2-4 times a day. Great for boosting your immune system and fighting viruses.

These natural remedies are discussed in more detail later in this guide. It is important to remember to check with you doctor before using any of these herbs as they may interfere with your current medication.

As stated earlier in this chapter, **HIV** – *Human Immunodeficiency Virus* – is currently one of the biggest emerging viruses that has caused an epidemic. It is a condition in humans that causes the immune system to progressively fail.

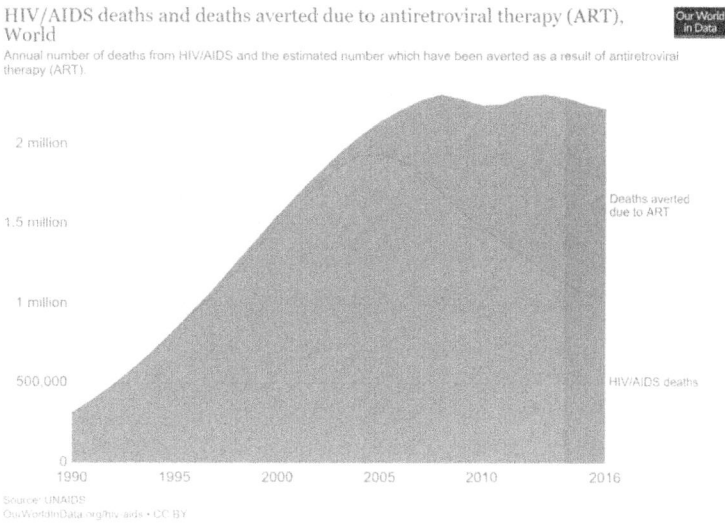

HIV/AIDS deaths and deaths averted due to antiretroviral therapy (ART), World

Annual number of deaths from HIV/AIDS and the estimated number which have been averted as a result of antiretroviral therapy (ART).

Although there is currently no cure for HIV, there are **antiretroviral medications** that have been specifically designed to stop the virus replicating within the body. They allow the body to repair itself and prevent further damage. There are possible side effects to this medication: nausea, diarrhea, skin rashes, sleep difficulties, etc., but the medication taken can be rearranged to change this.

Alongside the medication, doctors will recommend that HIV sufferers exercise, eat well, don't drink or smoke, and have a yearly flu shot to give their immune system the best chance possible.

There have also been a wide range of studies exploring the possibility of getting help from more natural, herbal remedies. A 2013 study published in the *African Journal of Traditional, Complementary, and Alternative Medicine* (http://www.greenmedinfo.com/blog/black-seed-completely-cures-hiv-case-study) has made the claim that **Black Seed Extract** (*Nigella sativa*) **used by an HIV patient resulted in a full recovery**, leaving them with no detectable HIV antibodies:

"Nigella sativa has been documented to possess many therapeutic functions in medicine but the least expected is sero-reversion in HIV infection which is very rare despite extensive therapy with highly active anti-retroviral therapy (HAART)."

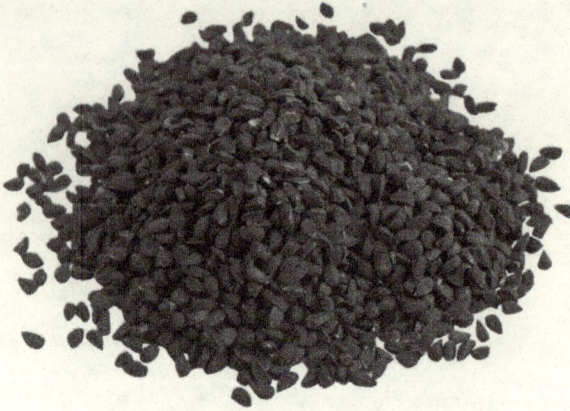

Other more natural remedies have been used by HIV patients to strengthen their immune systems, provide relief from the side effects from the traditional medicine, and give them a better quality of life. These include:

- *Immune System Therapies* – Designed to support the immune system. These include Ashwagandha, Astragalus, Atractylodes, Cat's Claw, Ginseng, Greater Celandine, Shatavari, Shiitake and Maitake Mushrooms.

- *Antimicrobial Therapies* – Designed to kill bacteria, viruses, and fungi. These include Garlic, Goldenseal, Neem, Propolis, Sanguinaria, Tea Tree.

- *Antioxidants* – Prevent the damage caused by our body's natural processes. These include Ginger, Ginkgo, Milk Thistle, Turmeric.

- *HIV-related Conditions* – There are some conditions caused by HIV. These natural remedies are used to combat them:
  - o   Greater Celandine to help with Kaposi's sarcoma.
  - o   Aloe Vera to help with skin issues.
  - o   Marijuana to help with wasting.
  - o   Lemon Balm to help with herpes simplex and insomnia.
  - o   Ginkgo to help with dementia.
  - o   St. John's Wort to help with moderate depression.

- *General Well-being* – Sometimes the herbs are used just to make HIV sufferers feel a little better. These can include Ashwagandha, Ginseng, Shatavari.

Ebola is another recent emergent virus that has a very high death rate, killing approximately 50% of its sufferers. The symptoms include fever, rash, sore throat, muscle pain, headaches. This all happens before the kidney and liver function of victims begins to decrease.

Ebola Outbreak in West Africa as of August 8, 2014

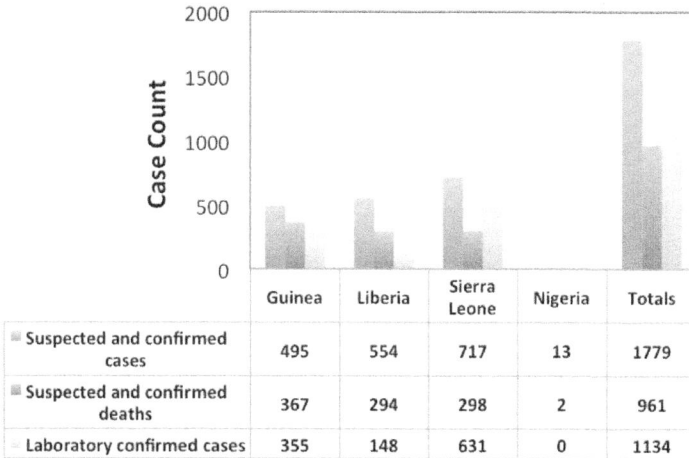

	Guinea	Liberia	Sierra Leone	Nigeria	Totals
Suspected and confirmed cases	495	554	717	13	1779
Suspected and confirmed deaths	367	294	298	2	961
Laboratory confirmed cases	355	148	631	0	1134

At this current time (in 2020), there aren't any licensed treatments or vaccines available for Ebola virus, although they are being worked on. However, there are treatments being used, such as blood products, immune therapies, and drug therapies.

There were two outbreaks of the Ebola virus in 1976, in Sudan and Democratic Republic of Congo simultaneously. The newest outbreak, which was first noted in March 2014, has lasted much longer and is much more of a threat. The most severely affected countries are Guinea, Sierra Leone, and Liberia, which are all lacking any resources due to recent periods of conflict and instability. The virus is spread by direct human contact and bodily fluids, so anyone suspected of suffering from the virus must be placed in isolated quarantine to prevent it from spreading any further.

Ebola Data (http://www.who.int/mediacentre/factsheets/fs103/en/):

Year	Country	Ebola Virus Species	Cases	Deaths	Fatality
2012	Democratic Republic of Congo	Bundibugyo	57	29	51%

2012	Uganda	Sudan	7	4	57%
2012	Uganda	Sudan	24	17	74%
2011	Uganda	Sudan	1	1	100%
2008	Democratic Republic of Congo	Zaire	32	14	44%
2007	Uganda	Bundibugyo	149	37	25%
2007	Democratic Republic of Congo	Zaire	264	187	71%
2005	Congo	Zaire	12	10	83%
2004	Sudan	Sudan	17	7	41%
2003 (Nov–Dec)	Congo	Zaire	35	29	83%
2003 (Jan–Apr)	Congo	Zaire	143	128	90%
2001–2002	Congo	Zaire	59	44	75%
2001–2002	Gabon	Zaire	65	53	82%
2000	Uganda	Sudan	425	224	53%
1996	South Africa (ex-Gabon)	Zaire	1	1	100%
1996 (Jul–Dec)	Gabon	Zaire	60	45	75%
1996 (Jan–Apr)	Gabon	Zaire	31	21	68%
1995	Democratic Republic of Congo	Zaire	315	254	81%
1994	Cote d'lvoire	Taï Forest	1	0	0%
1994	Gabon	Zaire	52	31	60%

1979	Sudan	Sudan	34	22	65%
1977	Democratic Republic of Congo	Zaire	1	1	100%
1976	Sudan	Sudan	284	151	53%
1976	Democratic Republic of Congo	Zaire	318	280	88%

According to some sources, magnesium salts, sodium bicarbonate, iodine, selenium, and Vitamin C are the key to resolving Ebola.

These more **natural remedies** have been proven in tests and studies to **help the human body fight and defend itself against other viral infections** – which suggests that they stand a very good chance at helping the victims of the Ebola virus.

The Zika Virus

This is yet another virus that came into the limelight after Ebola, in 2015. Its origin is traced to a mosquito in the genus Aedes, and was discovered in 1947 in Uganda.

Given that there have been many other diseases with similar symptoms to those of Zika, there was no special attention paid to this disease until 2015, when there was a serious outbreak in Brazil that ended in November 2016. Notably, there was increased evidence in 2015 that pointed to various infections with Zika that could cause neurological problems and serious birth defects, the most common of which being Microcephaly.

Transmission and data

While this virus can be spread from mother to child and through sexual activity, it's predominantly spread through Aedes albopictus and Aedes aegypti mosquitos.

When someone is infected, they start experiencing joint pain, rashes, red eyes, low grade fever and, sometimes, headache and muscle pain.

Here's a recent graphic representation of the number of territories that have reported Zika virus transmission.

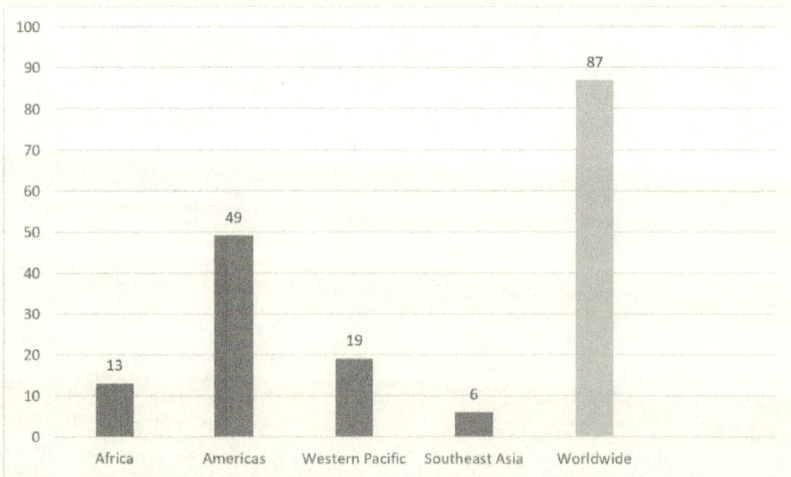

Here's a more detailed illustration of the number of territories with reported number of cases, and the total number of cases right from the onset.

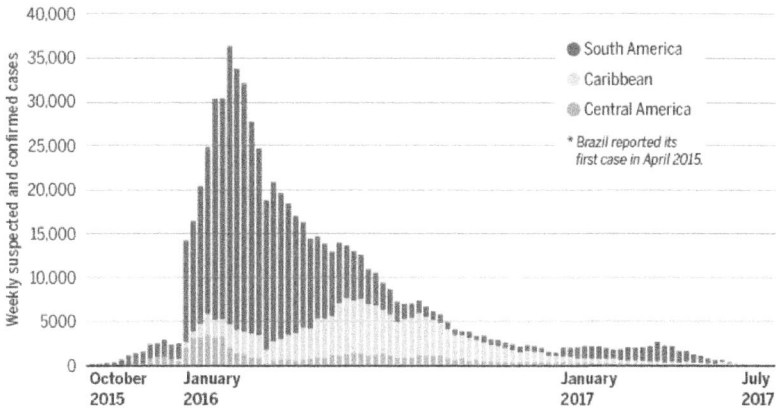

There is no known treatment for this virus, which means that there is a great need to prevent it. Based on the mode of transmission, the only way to prevent Zika virus is by avoiding mosquito bites if living in a high-risk area or if one is traveling to such areas.

What's more, if anyone finds themselves in those areas during their pregnancy, they should try to abstain until their doctor tells them otherwise, or use condoms each time they have sex.

The remedy

There is no Zika virus-specific treatment that has been found effective. Any treatment is meant to simply relieve symptoms – you combine rest, fluids, and medication to get relief. Specific medicine that has been found to help with this is acetaminophen (Tylenol, others) — these help to relieve the fever and the joint pain.

The best way to approach this disease is by strengthening the immune system by eating a lot of fruits and vegetables, drinking water, and relieving symptoms with rest. Even though some medications have been suggested for this purpose, such as above-mentioned acetaminophen, this disease is best approached naturally, with herbs such as basil, berberine, or turmeric.

Here are some of the studies confirming the effectiveness of plant remedies in the prevention and improvement of Zika virus:

One study at ncbi.nlm.nih.gov/pmc/articles/PMC6356660 confirms the use of:

- Berberine compound found in *Berberis vulgaris*. Beyond improving the symptoms of Zika and preventing the disease, this plant can also treat infections of the lower urinary tract and slow down the effects of other organisms including fungi and chlamydia bacteria.

- Emodin compound found in *Rheum palmatum (Chinese rhubarb), Polygonum multiflorum, Aloe vera, and Cassia obtusifolia (Chinese senna or sicklepod)*. This compound is mainly effective in respiratory illnesses by strengthening the immune system.

Another study at:
sciencedirect.com/science/article/pii/S0166354216307483 confirms the use of:

Curcumin, a component of turmeric. Curcumin is a great pain reliever especially in the joints and muscle areas.

The MERS-COV

The Middle East Respiratory Syndrome Coronavirus was first reported in Saudi Arabia in December 2012 and since then, about 2,400 cases have been confirmed in 27 countries. Though present in other parts of the world like Europe, America, and Africa, the most reported cases have been confirmed and reported from the Middle East.

While the source of the MERS-COV is still unknown, studies and the pattern of transmission point towards a type of camel, known as dromedary camels, in the Middle East as reservoirs of the virus, from which human beings became infected.

Most people diagnosed with this condition display symptoms like cough and fever, accompanied by severe pneumonia. When the condition becomes critical, the individual tends to display symptoms like acute respiratory distress syndrome (ARDS), renal failure, pericarditis, and disseminated intravascular coagulation (DIC).

Transmission and data

This virus can be transmitted from one person to another, and it's believed this happens through droplets (usually from coughing), which are the main mode of transmission. It's important to note that medical officers still don't understand exactly how this virus is transmitted.

All the reported cases have been connected to the countries within or close to the Arabian Peninsula. Most of the reported infections are in people who either traveled from the Arabian Peninsula before they became sick or people who lived in that region. A few contracted MERS after being in close contact with the infected persons (who had traveled from the Arabian Peninsula recently).

Notably, the biggest outbreak of this disease outside the Arabian Peninsula took place in the Republic of Korea in 2015 and was related with a traveler who had returned from the Arabian Peninsula.

Here's the most recent data on the reported cases in Saudi Arabia and other affected countries since 2012.

	Country	Cumulative number of confirmed MERS-CoV human cases	First observation	Last Observation
Middle East	Saudi Arabia	2 129	13/06/2012	**17/02/2020**
	United Arab Emirates	91	19/03/2013	**18/12/2019**
	Jordan	28	02/04/2012	26/09/2015
	Qatar	22	15/08/2013	29/11/2019
	Oman	24	26/10/2013	20/02/2019
	Iran (Islamic Republic of)	6	11/05/2014	18/03/2015
	Kuwait	4	30/10/2013	08/09/2015
	Lebanon	2	22/04/2014	08/06/2017
	Yemen	1	17/03/2014	17/03/2014
	Bahrain (the Kingdom of)	1	04/04/2016	04/04/2016
Europe	United Kingdom	5	03/09/2012	16/08/2018
	Germany	3	05/10/2012	07/03/2015
	Netherlands	2	01/05/2014	05/05/2014
	France	2	23/04/2013	27/04/2013
	Austria	2	22/09/2014	08/09/2016
	Turkey	1	25/09/2014	25/09/2014
	Italy	1	25/05/2013	25/05/2013
	Greece	1	08/04/2014	08/04/2014
Asia	Republic of Korea	186	11/05/2015	28/08/2018
	Philippines	2	15/04/2014	30/06/2015
	Thailand	3	10/06/2015	25/07/2016
	China	1	21/05/2015	21/05/2015
	Malaysia	2	08/04/2014	24/12/2017
Americas	United States of America	2	14/04/2014	01/05/2014
Africa	Tunisia	3	01/05/2013	17/06/2013
	Algeria	2	23/05/2014	23/05/2014
	Egypt	1	22/04/2014	22/04/2014

The remedy

There is no vaccine or specific treatment recommended for this disease. Therefore, infected people often get medical care that is largely meant to relieve the symptoms. For the severe cases, though, current treatment involves care for the support of the vital organ functions.

People are advised, however, to reduce their risk of contracting the MERS illness by taking the following precautionary measures:

- Washing hands often with soap and water – for at least 20 seconds per session. Alcohol-based hand sanitizers are also recommended as viable alternatives.

- Covering the mouth and nose with a tissue when sneezing or coughing, and then safely dumping the tissue in the trash.

- Avoiding touching the eyes, mouth, and nose with unwashed hands.

- Avoiding personal contact like kissing or sharing eating utensils with sick people.

- Cleaning and disinfecting frequently touched surfaces and objects like doorknobs.

You can also boost your immune system with herbs and other natural remedies, a method that has, over time, been proven to be more superior to drugs and many other preventive measures.

44 Ways to Strengthen an Immune System

1. Avoid Alcohol or Sugar
2. Barley Juice Powder
3. Beets
4. CBD
5. Celery Juice
6. Chaga Mushroom
7. Cinnamon
8. Colloidal Silver
9. Dancing
10. Drinking enough Water
11. Eating Organic Fruits & Veggies
12. Elderberry Syrup
13. Excersize
14. Exposure to Healthy Bacteria
15. Fermented Food
16. Fresh Air
17. Getting Enough Rest
18. Ginger
19. Healthy Sexual Activity
20. Healthy Soups
21. Intermittent Fasting
22. Juice Cleanse
23. Kissing
24. Kombucha
25. Lemons
26. Lions Mane Mushroom
27. Meditation
28. Nature Hikes
29. Olive Leaf Extract
30. Onion
31. Oregano Oil
32. Probiotics
33. Raw Garlic
34. Raw Honey
35. Reishi Mushroom
36. Selenium
37. Sunshine
38. Switching Between Hot & Cold Showers Intermittently
39. Teaspoon of Apple Cider Vinegar
40. Turkey Tail Mushroom
41. Turmeric Powder
42. Vitamins C & D
43. Wim Hof Breathing Technique
44. Zinc

Below are some studies confirming the effectiveness of plant remedies in the prevention and improvement of MERS-COV:

A study at <u>researchsquare.com/article/rs-15282/v2</u> confirms the use of:

Echinacea purpurea in the prophylactic treatment of all coronaviruses, including MERS-COV.

Another study at <u>ncbi.nlm.nih.gov/pubmed/24520776</u> confirms the use of:

Triterpenoid, a compound found in Licorice, in the treatment of MERS-COV.

Avian Influenza A (H7N9)

Avian influenza A is a subtype of influenza viruses, which were detected in birds in the past. Before it was found in China in 2013, this particular virus had not been previously seen in people or animals.

Beyond China, infected cases have been reported in Canada and Malaysia, which have so far totaled to 1,568 – out of which, 616 people have died since February 2013.

When a person becomes infected, they develop headaches, fever, and a cough, as well as breathing problems and muscle pain. Afterwards, the individual may experience pneumonia along with acute respiratory distress syndrome, multi-organ dysfunction, blood infection, muscle breakdown, and brain disease.

It's important to note that 40% of the infected cases died during the first four seasonal epidemics, but in total, nearly 20% of all people who've had contact with the infected animals have died. Ironically, the H7N9 doesn't normally affect human beings, as it is a bird flu virus. The virus, however, mutated or changed over time to affect humans, and given the fact that humans don't have immunity to new viruses, it makes sense as to why the H7N9 has been said to be very dangerous.

Transmission and data

Here's a detailed illustration of the number of infections recorded as of August 2018.

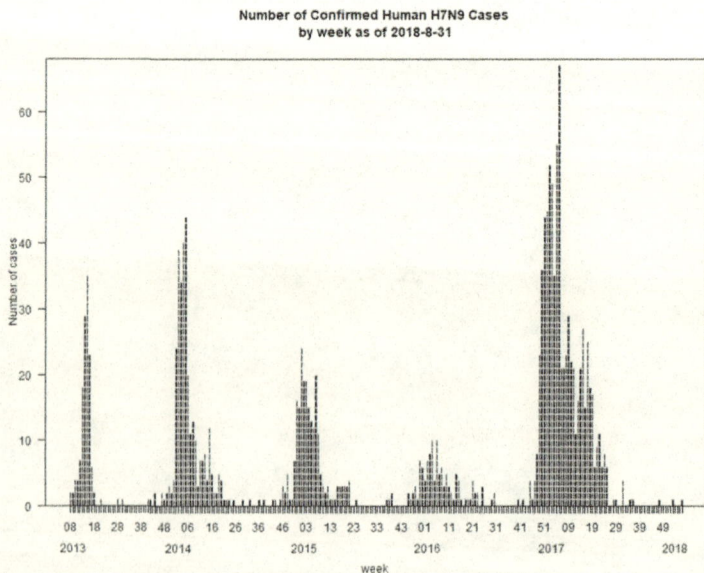

Number of Confirmed Human H7N9 Cases by week as of 2018-8-31

The virus is spread when birds shed the virus in their mucus or droppings, and a person makes contact with these products – whether the bird is alive or dead. The person contracts the virus when, for example, they then touch their mouth or eyes.

According to the Centers for Disease Control and Prevention (CDC), the virus can also travel through the air, for instance, as the bird flaps its wings – even if the bird doesn't appear to be ill.

The remedy

As with most novel viruses, there is no vaccine or a single treatment for H7N9, and the treatments offered to the affected patients are the existing antiviral drugs used to treat the common seasonal flu viruses. A class of drugs known as neuraminidase inhibitors is often used for such cases, even though they aren't effective in all people suffering from N7H9.

Everyone should, however, ensure they make steps to improve their immunity, which is best done with herbs and other natural remedies.

An example of the studies confirming the effectiveness of plant remedies in the prevention and improvement of A(H7N9):

This study at nature.com/articles/cr2014130 confirms the use of:

MIR2911 compound found in Honeysuckle Flower to treat A (H7N9).

Medical experts also propose the following precautionary measures to prevent infection:

- If you live in or travel to the high-risk areas, avoid touching birds and other animals like pigs.
- Only eat food (especially meat) that's cooked fully, not pink.
- Be meticulous about hand hygiene and general cleanliness.
- If you feel sick during or after your trip to a high-risk area, see a doctor.

<u>Covid-19 (Novel Coronavirus)</u>

At the time of this writing (March 2020), the World Health Organization had already declared the Covid-19's outbreak a pandemic. This was at a time when the virus had over 800,000 confirmed cases and over 40,000 deaths reported in 114 countries and territories spanning 6 continents since the virus came into the limelight in December 2019.

Most of the infections and deaths have occurred in mainland China, where 60 million people had been put under lockdown in efforts to contain the virus. Other countries among the greatest number of cases and deaths from the virus are United States, Spain, Italy, France, Germany, Iran, and others.

Here are the statistics in China.

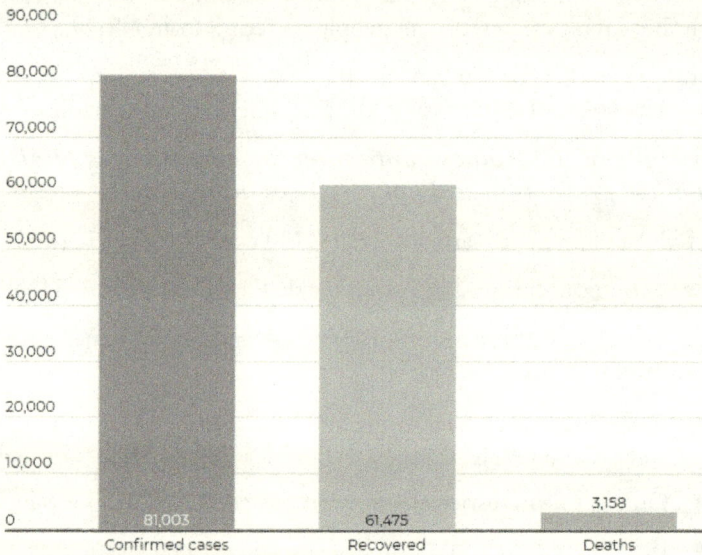

Other countries and regions affected are illustrated in the image below (with severity levels).

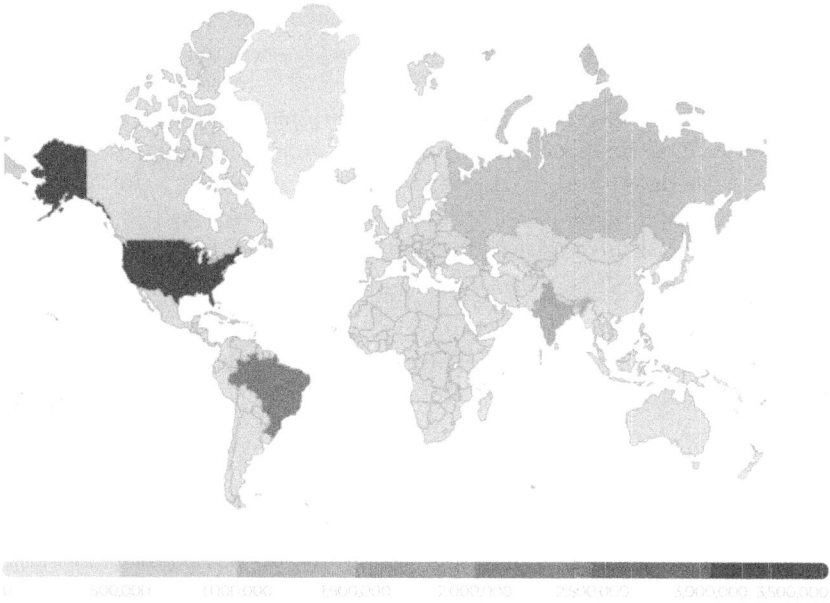

Territories with confirmed cases of Covid-19 as of July 22, 2020

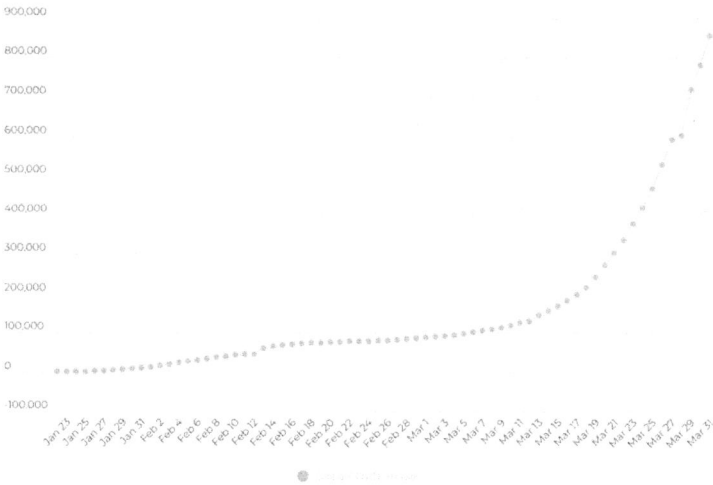

Coronavirus around the world

Transmission and data

Covid-19 is a coronavirus that is transmitted between animals and people. The animal source of this virus is still not clear, but experts speculate that bats may be its host and the virus gets passed to humans through other animal species, like the pangolin.

Just like the other coronaviruses, the Novel Coronavirus is usually transmitted from person to person through droplets when the infected person sneezes, coughs, or breathes out. Covid-19 can also be spread through contaminated surfaces like railings or door handles harboring the droplets. Recent studies indicate that Covid-19 lives on surfaces for different amounts of time, depending on material: copper – less than 4 hours, cardboard – up to 24 hours, steel or plastic – up to 72 hours. This makes it highly infectious, with specialists estimating that, on average, one carrier passes it on to 2-3 people.

When a person contracts this virus, they start displaying certain symptoms including dry cough, fever or fatigue. In more critical cases, the infection can lead to multi-organ failure, severe pneumonia, and death.

Luckily, the disease is mild in over 80% of cases, severe in 13%, and critical in only 6%.

Note that this disease is seen to be more severe in people with underlying medical conditions, such as diabetes, high blood pressure, and heart disease, or people with compromised lungs and other organs (who, in most cases, are the elderly).

The remedy

- The best way to prevent this disease is by practicing good hygiene, which includes good hand-washing practices (and hand sanitizing) each time an individual touches surfaces (like rails, poles, doors, etc.) in public spaces, and avoiding unnecessary face-touching in public (unless the hands are sanitized).

- Consider that the coronavirus can stay within the air for hours and up to one or more days on some surfaces, like cardboards and plastic. Ethanol, sodium hypochlorite, hydrogen peroxide, and other disinfectants have been seen to have viable effects on getting rid of the virus.

  TIP: to create a hand sanitizer at home, you can mix 3 parts of coconut oil with 1 part of concentrated olive oil.

- People should avoid close contact with other people they suspect are sick, or if they suspect themselves to be sick.

- It's important to cover the nose and mouth when sneezing and dispose of the used tissues safely.

- Use of face masks is also important for people who suspect themselves to be infected.

Even with all these measures, it's always prudent for everyone to keep their immune system strong and healthy as this the last line of defense.

Building your immune system

There is always a satisfying feeling a person gets in the face of danger — when the startling thought about their safety crosses their mind, and then they remember that they've taken the right measures to protect themselves from it. The nature and impact of the new coronavirus around the globe would make that feeling even more overwhelming.

An outbreak like this one is also a good way to give everyone the perfect chance to review how well they're caring for their bodies, and particularly the steps they're taking to keep themselves immune to all kinds of infection.

So, generally, *good self-care should include*:

- Staying well-hydrated (drink plenty of water).
- Getting enough rest and trying to reduce stress.
- Supporting your lungs by taking a break from smoking.
- Plenty of sunlight on your skin and in your eyes.
- Spending time in fresh air (deep breathing/walks in nature).
- Treating food as medication and therefore focusing on eating a rainbow of vegetables and fruits every day. It's important to ensure half of our food intake consists of fruits and vegetables. Try to avoid excessive sugar.

However, a consistent intake of fruits and vegetables should be treated as a baseline. Besides other nutrients, it's good to boost healthy food sources with a bit **more vitamin C**. While many studies have confirmed the efficacy of this nutrient in strengthening the immune system against viral infections, including SARS and pneumonia, an advanced complication of coronavirus, most of us are already familiar with its effectiveness — especially in combating and preventing viral respiratory tract infections. So, take several grams per day and build up the dose gradually to prevent negative side effects.

There are many herbal remedies that can give you a good daily dose of vitamin C, including:

- *Garlic* – any person at high risk of contracting the virus should aim for 2-3 cloves per day (consumed as part of regular meals); otherwise, 1 clove is ideal – at the absolute minimum.
- *Ginger* – this spice contains 5 milligrams of vitamin C per 100 grams. It has a long tradition of being used for its anti-

inflammatory and antioxidant effects, as well as its immune-boosting benefits. A quarter inch of fresh ginger per day is enough to provide protection against a host of viruses, including the Novel Coronavirus.

Other equally useful natural remedies for the immune system include:

- Echinacea
- Elderberry – for prevention and building immunity
- Green tea – considered helpful during SARS breakout
- Turmeric
- Colloidal silver
- NAC – highly recommended for Covid-19 virus, supports lungs and breaks up mucus
- Kyolic Aged Garlic Extract (Immune formula)

Beyond the aforementioned, **here are some of the other herbs confirmed by research (**at ncbi.nlm.nih.gov/pubmed/32065348**) to prevent or improve Covid-19**:

- *Radix glycyrrhizae (Gancao)*
- *Rhizoma Atractylodis Macrocephalae (Baizhu)*
- *Fructus forsythia (Lianqiao)*
- *Radix astragali (Huangqi)*
- *Lonicerae Japonicae Flos (Jinyinhua)*
- *Radix saposhnikoviae (Fangfeng)*

NOTE – If anyone suspects themselves of having contracted a coronavirus infection, they should:

- Call their general practitioner for advice.
- Continue boosting their immunity with natural remedies.
- Keep a safe distance between themselves and other people, and encourage people around them to wash their hands as often as possible.
- Avoid taking ibuprofen, aspirin, naproxen, or other forms of NSAIDs since these suppress immunity and facilitate the spread of the virus.
- Avoid eating sugary foods since they lower the immune function.
- Avoid panicking as they follow the steps above carefully.

A virus's lifecycle includes:

1. *Adsorption*: Virus particle binds to host cell.

2. *Entry*: Virus infects the cell by fusing its own oily membrane with that of the healthy cell. Once inside, it begins releasing a bit of its genetic material known as the ribonucleic acid, or RNA.

3. The infected cell starts reading the RNA immediately and making proteins that will ensure the immune system is kept at bay. It does so also to assist assemble new copies of the virus.

4. *Replication*: As the infection progresses, the cell machinery is used to churn out fresh spikes and other proteins to form more copies of the virus.

5. *Assembly*: The new virus copies are then assembled and taken to the outer areas of the cell.

6. *Release*: The infected cell releases millions of copies of the virus and then the cell breaks down and dies. The virus copies then infect nearby cells.

In the case of Covid-19, the virus may end up in droplets that are expelled out of the lungs, and then cause fever as the immune system struggles to clear the virus. This may progress to an extent that the immune system starts attacking the lung cells. The resulting fluid and dead cells may block different areas within the lungs, leading to difficulties in breathing.

The key to any emerging virus is to find a way to cure it before it becomes an epidemic. As shown by the current examples of these – in particular HIV and Ebola – it is virtually impossible to do this as it takes years of study, testing, and quality control to get these medications on the market, and even then, they often provide undesirable side effects. Herbal remedies give sufferers an immediately available alternative to this, which should be considered by doctors and patients.

GLOBAL OUTBREAKS
Worst epidemics in recent history

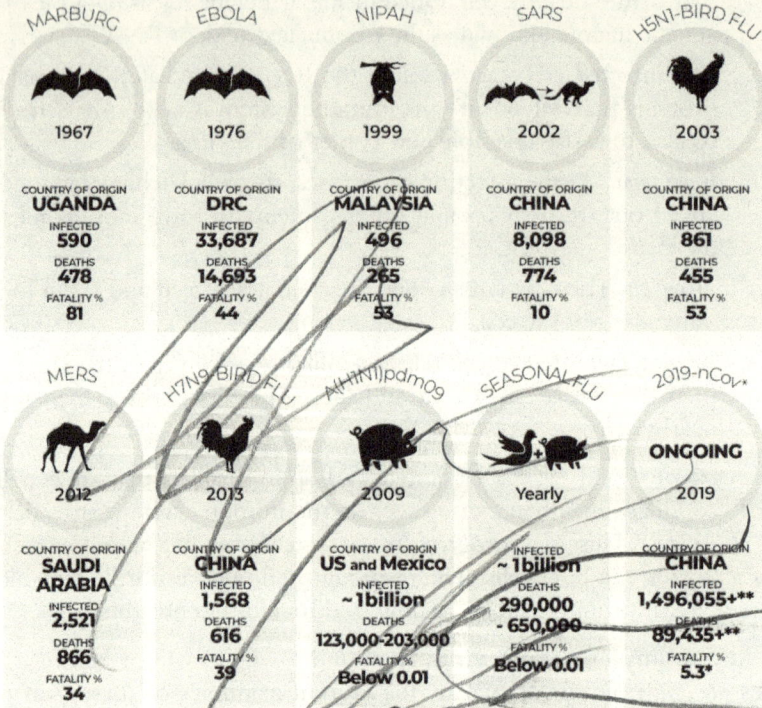

MARBURG

1967

COUNTRY OF ORIGIN
UGANDA
INFECTED
590
DEATHS
478
FATALITY %
81

EBOLA

1976

COUNTRY OF ORIGIN
DRC
INFECTED
33,687
DEATHS
14,693
FATALITY %
44

NIPAH

1999

COUNTRY OF ORIGIN
MALAYSIA
INFECTED
496
DEATHS
265
FATALITY %
53

SARS

2002

COUNTRY OF ORIGIN
CHINA
INFECTED
8,098
DEATHS
774
FATALITY %
10

H5N1-BIRD FLU

2003

COUNTRY OF ORIGIN
CHINA
INFECTED
861
DEATHS
455
FATALITY %
53

MERS

2012

COUNTRY OF ORIGIN
SAUDI ARABIA
INFECTED
2,521
DEATHS
866
FATALITY %
34

H7N9-BIRD FLU

2013

COUNTRY OF ORIGIN
CHINA
INFECTED
1,568
DEATHS
616
FATALITY %
39

A(H1N1)pdm09

2009

COUNTRY OF ORIGIN
US and Mexico
INFECTED
~ 1 billion
DEATHS
123,000-203,000
FATALITY %
Below 0.01

SEASONAL FLU

Yearly

INFECTED
~ 1 billion
DEATHS
290,000 - 650,000
FATALITY %
Below 0.01

2019-nCoV*

ONGOING

2019

COUNTRY OF ORIGIN
CHINA
INFECTED
1,496,055+**
DEATHS
89,435+**
FATALITY %
5.3*

*Origins yet to be determined
**Approximate figures as of April 8, 2020

Source: WHO | JOHNS HOPKINS UNIVERSITY | Last updated: 11:30 GMT, April 8, 2020   @AJLabs ALJAZEERA

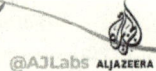

CHAPTER 2
EYE-OPENING ALTERNATIVE MEDICINE STATISTICS

The National Center for Complementary and Integrative Health (NCCIH) is an agency within the US government that conducts research about complementary and alternative medicine. They have conducted a lot of research (http://nccam.nih.gov) into the usage of complementary and alternative medicine.

The diagrams below show the findings of this data (CAM = *Complementary and Alternative Medicine*).

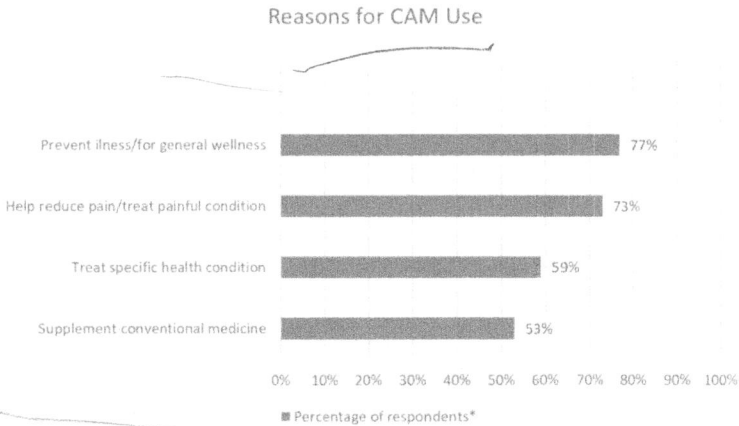

Reasons for CAM Use

Reason	Percentage
Prevent ilness/for general wellness	77%
Help reduce pain/treat painful condition	73%
Treat specific health condition	59%
Supplement conventional medicine	53%

0% 10% 20% 30% 40% 50% 60% 70% 80% 90% 100%

■ Percentage of respondents*

*Base: Respondents who used CAM in past 12 months or ever (n=539). Sampling error = 4.2 percentage points. Respondents could choose more than one answer.

Source: AARP/NCCAM Survey of U.S. Adults 50+, 2010

Type of CAM Used in the Past 12 Months

Category	Percentage
Herbal products or dietary supplements	37%
Massage therapy, chiropractic manipulation, other bodyword	22%
Mind/body practices	9%
Naturopathy, acupuncture, homeopathy	5%
Other types	1%

■ Percentage of respondents*

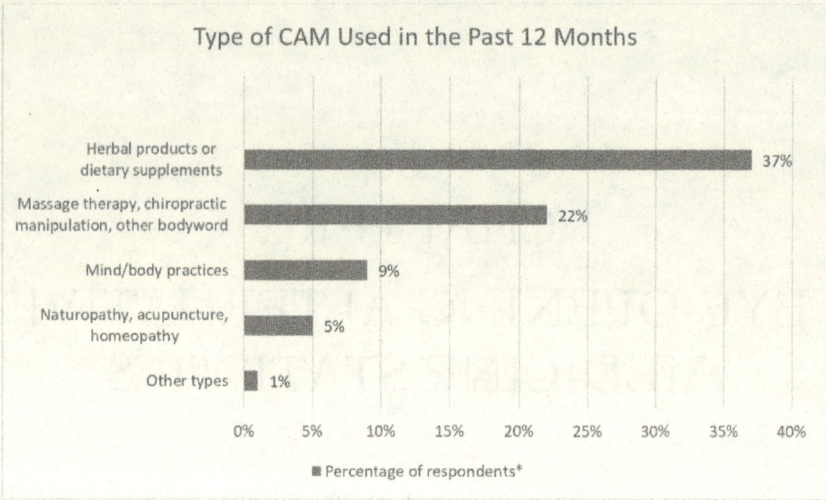

*Base: All respondents (n=1013). Sampling error = 3.1 percentage points. Respondents could choose more than one answer.

Source: AARP/NCCAM Survey of U.S. Adults 50+, 2010

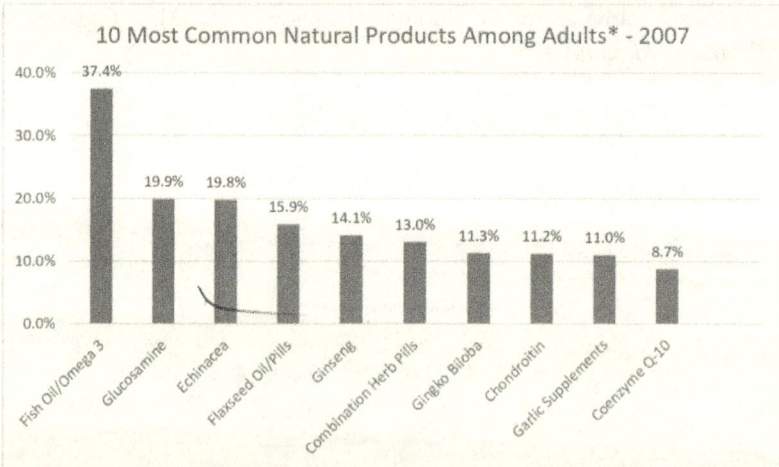

10 Most Common Natural Products Among Adults* - 2007

Product	Percentage
Fish Oil/Omega 3	37.4%
Glucosamine	19.9%
Echinacea	19.8%
Flaxseed Oil/Pills	15.9%
Ginseng	14.1%
Combination Herb Pills	13.0%
Gingko Biloba	11.3%
Chondroitin	11.2%
Garlic Supplements	11.0%
Coenzyme Q-10	8.7%

*Percentages among adults who used natural products in the last 30 days.

Source: Barnes PM, Bloom B, Nahin R. CDC National Health Statistics Report #12. Complementary and Alternative Medicine Use Among Adults and Children: United States, 2007.

Out-of-Pocket Costs for Selected CAM Therapies*

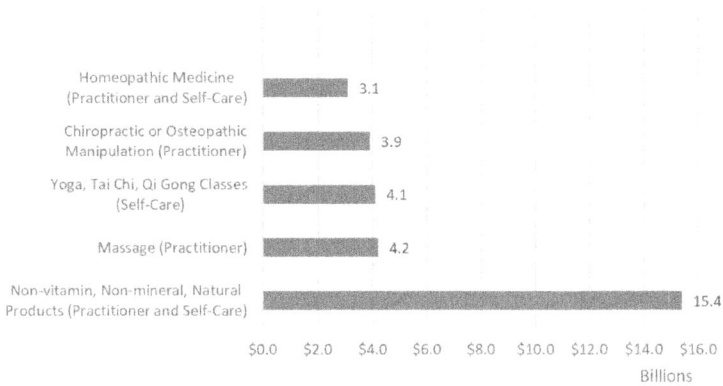

Therapy	Billions
Homeopathic Medicine (Practitioner and Self-Care)	3.1
Chiropractic or Osteopathic Manipulation (Practitioner)	3.9
Yoga, Tai Chi, Qi Gong Classes (Self-Care)	4.1
Massage (Practitioner)	4.2
Non-vitamin, Non-mineral, Natural Products (Practitioner and Self-Care)	15.4

Totals for non-vitamin, non-mineral, natural products and homeopathy include both — CAM practitioner costs and costs of purchasing CAM products. Totals for massage and chiropractic manipulation are only for CAM practitioner costs. Totals for yoga, tai chi and qi gong classes are only the costs of purchasing CAM products.

CAM Use by U.S. Adults and Children

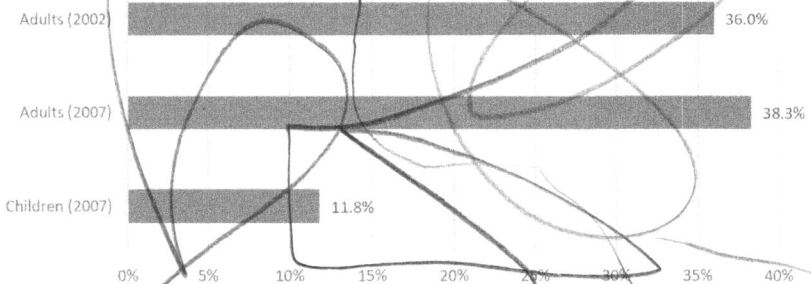

Group	Percentage
Adults (2002)	36.0%
Adults (2007)	38.3%
Children (2007)	11.8%

Source: Barnes PM, Bloom B, Nahin R. CDC National Health Statistics Report #12. Complementary and Alternative Medicine Use Among Adults and Children: United States, 2007.

Use of Complementary Health Approaches in the U.S.
National Health Interview Survey (NHIS)

Diseases/conditions for which complementaryhealth approaches are most frequently used among children—2012

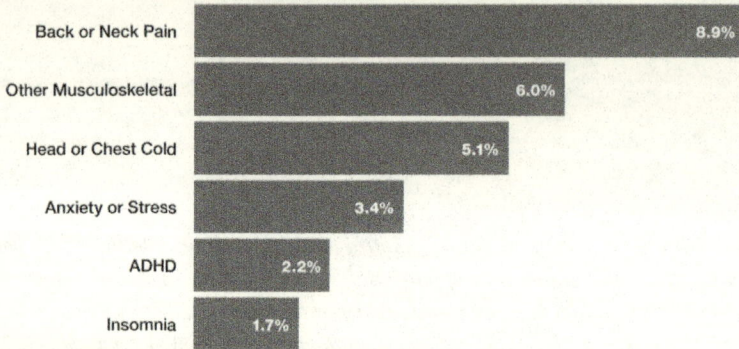

Condition	Percentage
Back or Neck Pain	8.9%
Other Musculoskeletal	6.0%
Head or Chest Cold	5.1%
Anxiety or Stress	3.4%
ADHD	2.2%
Insomnia	1.7%

*Dietary supplements other than vitamins and minerals.

Citation: Black LI, Clarke TC, Barnes PM, Stussman BJ, Nahin RL. Use of complementary health approaches among children aged 4-17 years in the United States: National Health Interview Survey, 2007-2012. National health statistics reports: no 78. Hyattsville, MD: National Center for Health Statistics. 2015.

From this data, it's easy to see the benefits of herbal medication and why more people are turning to it on an annual basis. The NCCAM data below shows the age range of people using complementary and alternative medicine, and based on all the information shown so far, this is projected to continue to grow dramatically.

Alternative Medicine

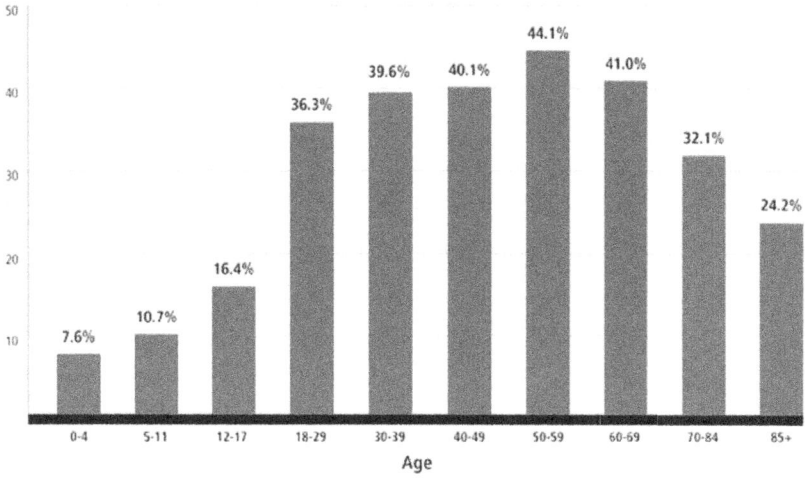

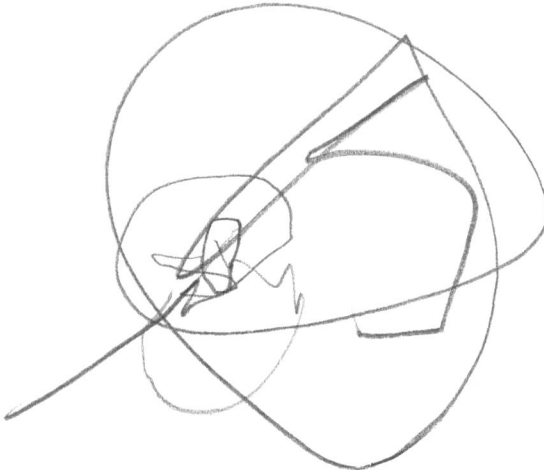

CHAPTER 3
USAGE OF ANTIVIRALS – ALL YOU NEED TO KNOW

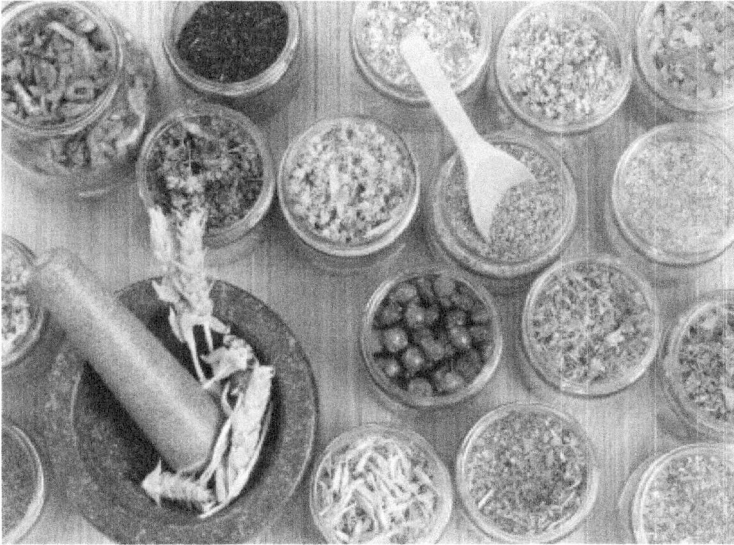

There are many reasons why people make the change to herbal medication, and in particular antivirals, but of course, you need to be sure that the choice is right for you. *A study (http://umm.edu/health/medical/altmed/treatment/herbal-medicine) shows* that **nearly one third of Americans already use herbal remedies** and intend to continue to do so, but everyone needs to *take the following conditions into consideration*:

- *Other medication that you are taking* – You will need to consult with your doctor to check that there will be no negative interactions.

- *Side effects* – Although herbal medication **has a smaller possibility** of side effects than conventional antibiotics, **you still need to be aware of what *could* occur.**

- *Regulation* – Herbal medication isn't regulated in the way that conventional treatments are. There are a lot of resources and information available for you to make your own decisions, but **there are a few groups that haven't been properly tested on** – women who are pregnant or breastfeeding, children, or the elderly. It is always best to consult with your doctor first.

A virus is described as:

"Any of a large group of submicroscopic infective agents that are regarded either as extremely simple microorganisms or as extremely complex molecules, that typically contain a protein coat surrounding an RNA or DNA core of genetic material but no semipermeable membrane, that are capable of growth and multiplication only in living cells, and that cause various important diseases in humans, animals, or plants."

A virus is not considered 'live' as it cannot replicate outside of a host. Viruses enter and infect cells before using them to replicate and mutate, which can eventually kill the cells. An example of this is the influenza virus, which attacks the respiratory system.

It's difficult to produce prescription antiviral medication that is safe and effective without damaging the cell that the virus has used to replicate. The first experimental antivirals were developed in the 1960s through trial-and-error discovery methods, targeting the herpes virus initially. It wasn't until the 1980s, when the full genetic sequences of viruses were understood, that scientists could work out the right chemicals needed to thwart their reproductive cycle.

"Antiviral medicines work by biochemically making it impossible for the virus to replicate," explains Randy Wexler, MD, assistant professor of family medicine at the Ohio State University College of Medicine in Columbus.

Below is a list of **the most commonly prescribed antiviral medications**:

Generic	Brand Name
Acyclovir	*Zovirax, Sitavig*
Famciclovir	*Famvir*
Penciclovir	*Denavir*
Valacyclovir	*Valtrex*
Trifluridine	*Viroptic*
Docosanol	*Abreva*

Generic	Brand Name
Adamantane Derivatives	
Amantadine	*Symmetrel*
Rimantadine	*Flumadine*
Neuraminidase Inhibitors	
Oseltamivir	*Tamiflu*
Zanamivir	*Relenze*

The Way Herbal Antivirals Work

Antivirals work by boosting the processes of the immune system. For instance, antivirals can disrupt the viral replication cycle by binding to specific enzymes and preventing adsorption of a host cell.

Michael Moore, an herbalist, describes antivirals in his medical glossary as:

"An agent that experimentally inhibits the proliferation and viability of infectious viruses. In our domain of herbal medicines, some plants will slow or inhibit the adsorption or random initial attachment of viruses, extend the lifespan of infected target cells, or speed up several aspects of immunity, including complement, antibody, and phagocytosis responses. Herbal antivirals work best on respiratory viruses such as influenza, adenoviruses, rhinoviruses, and the enteric echoviruses. Touted as useful in the alphabet group of slow viruses (HIV, EBV, CMV, etc.), they really help to limit secondary concurrent respiratory infections that often accompany immunosuppression."

Of course, **there are pros and cons to both traditional and herbal antivirals**. These are examined below:

Traditional Antivirals

Pros:

- They help you get over the viral infection faster.
- They are easy to take – often coming in the form of tablets or capsules.
- Traditional medication is regulated by a governing body to ensure its safety.

Cons:

- Side effects include nausea, vomiting, cough, runny/stuffy nose, diarrhea.
- They aren't essential. You will recover from the viral infection without them.

Herbal Antivirals

Pros:

- Herbal antivirals offer far fewer side effects.
- They cost much less.
- They are far more easily available.

Cons:

- There is a lack of regulation in herbal antivirals, which means it can be more difficult to find all the information you need.
- They can interact with other medication you're taking.

There are **many ways that your body can fight infections and strengthen your immune system naturally** – it is designed to do so. Sometimes it just needs a little help when it comes to viruses. Aside from herbal medication, there are factors that you can include in your everyday lifestyle as preventative methods:

- Avoid contracting infections by practicing hygiene and clean food preparation.
- Maintain healthy blood pressure.
- Eat healthy foods such as vegetables, whole grains, fruits, and foods low in saturated fats.
- Control your weight with regular exercise.
- Quit smoking, and only drink alcohol in moderation.
- Be sure to get plenty of sleep.
- Complete medical screenings appropriate for your age and potential health risks.

There are many *essential oils that contain antiviral properties*.

The following 5 are the most popular: *Clove, Oregano, Basil, Cinnamon,* and *Peppermint.*

CHAPTER 4

BEST SOURCES FOR HERBAL ANTIVIRALS

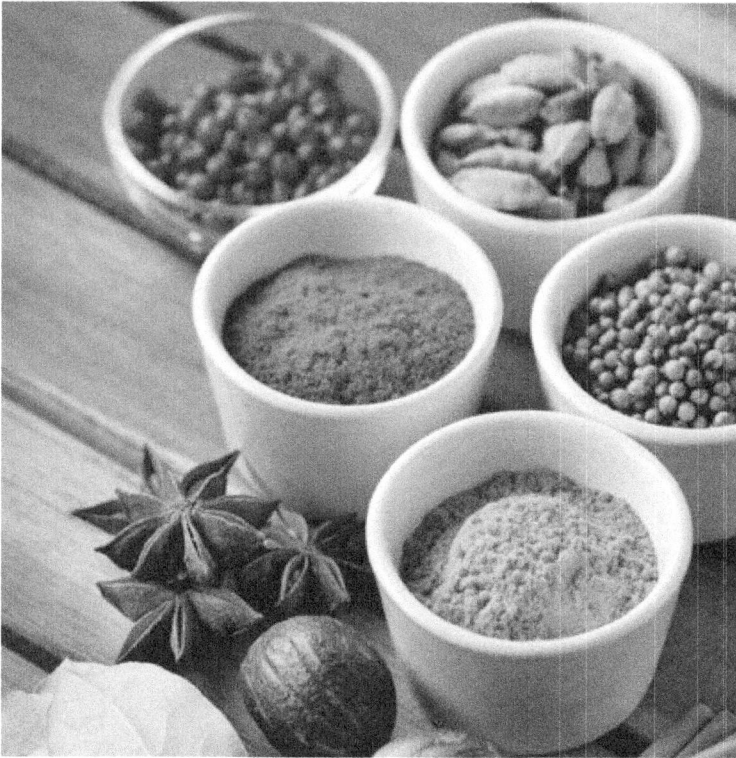

Herbal antivirals can be found everywhere. They don't necessarily have to be purchased in supplement form. In fact, including **antiviral food** in your everyday diet is a great way to help prevent viruses from affecting you.

These are considered the **Top natural antivirals in foods, herbs, and spices**:

- Cat's Claw
- Cranberry
- Elderberry
- Ginger
- Lemon Balm
- Licorice Root
- Olive Leaf
- Oregano
- Green Tea

These are suggested to be the **Best antiviral herbs**:

- Turmeric
- Cinnamon
- Garlic
- Oregano
- Rosemary
- Ginger
- Peppermint
- Basil
- Echinacea
- Pau D'arco
- St. John's Wort

CHAPTER 5
TOP 45 ANTIVIRAL HERBS

1. Garlic

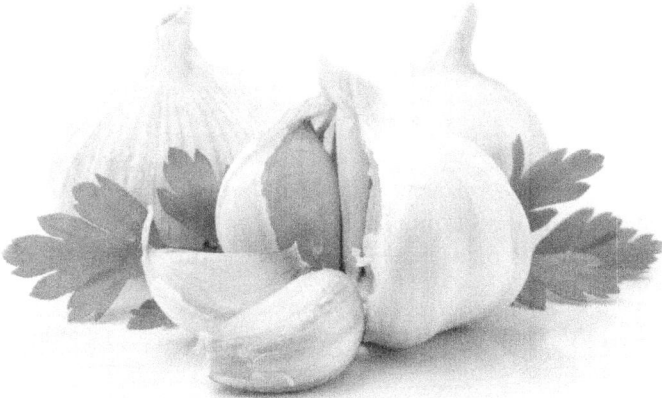

Garlic has been considered a folk remedy in various cultures and is used to protect against influenza and colds. This herb has been cultivated since the days of the pharaohs, over 5,000 years, and trusted due to its medicinal properties for just as long. Various lab studies have found that Garlic possesses antifungal, antiviral, and antibacterial properties. Its multitude of beneficial compounds, such as allicin and various sulfur compounds, are the key to Garlic's healing properties. Allicin is the most significant compound, which is responsible for Garlic's distinct odor. It is generated by the compound alliin when fresh Garlic is broken down, either by chewing or chopping. Powdered supplements with allicin potential can also be a good source. However, aged Garlic products will lack allicin, but the s-allyl cysteine compound may counteract that lack. Garlic has been known to combat strains of the influenza virus, types I and II of the herpes simplex virus, and the common cold.

TIP: If you are worried about the bad odor of Garlic, try eating parsley after. It is known to eliminate the strong odor. Also if you want to preserve Garlic's anticancer properties, cut 1 clove and leave it for 10 minutes before cooking! Alliinase enzyme produces allyl sulfur, a cancer fighting compound, in those 10 minutes.

Availability: Can be purchased from most food-based shops. (e.g. naturesbest.co.uk, iHerb.com, Amazon.com)

Antiviral Properties: Allicin is the most powerful antiviral compound in Garlic. This sulfur compound is *primarily used to fight the cold virus*.

Collection & Preparation: Available as a powder, tablets, capsules, a tincture or can be consumed in food (preferably raw). Also look for aged Garlic extract, which is known to increase the bioavailability of Garlic in the body.

Dosage: *For respiratory infections* – 2-5 g of Garlic in dried bulb form or 2-4 mL of Garlic alcoholic extract taken by mouth 3 times daily.

Possible Side Effects: The smell can often lead to bad breath, heartburn, and upset stomach.

Contraindications: Do not take if allergic to Garlic; people with sensitive skin or mouth/tongue problems should avoid external use of Garlic. Do not take high doses during pregnancy or while breastfeeding. Avoid taking it with anticoagulants or diabetes medication and if you're planning a surgery within the next 7 days.

Alternatives: All close relatives of onions and Garlic, including shallots, leeks, chive, and rakkyo.

Other Uses: Blood Pressure, Digestion, Asthma, Cough, Infections, Stomach Ulcers, Cancer, Blood Clotting, Impotence, Arthritis, Antiseptic.

Garlic, raw

Nutritional value per 100 g (3.5 oz)

Energy	623 kJ (149 kcal)

Carbohydrates	33.06 g
Sugars	1 g
Dietary fiber	2.1 g

Fat	0.5 g

Protein	6.36 g

Vitamins	Quantity	%DV[†]
Thiamine (B$_1$)	0.2 mg	17%
Riboflavin (B$_2$)	0.11 mg	9%
Niacin (B$_3$)	0.7 mg	5%
Pantothenic acid (B$_5$)	0.596 mg	12%
Vitamin B$_6$	1.2350 mg	95%
Folate (B$_9$)	3 µg	1%
Choline	23.2 mg	5%
Vitamin C	31.2 mg	38%

Minerals	Quantity	%DV[†]
Calcium	181 mg	18%
Iron	1.7 mg	13%
Magnesium	25 mg	7%
Manganese	1.672 mg	80%
Phosphorus	153 mg	22%
Potassium	401 mg	9%
Sodium	17 mg	1%
Zinc	1.16 mg	12%

Other constituents	Quantity
Water	59 g
selenium	14.2 µg

2. Echinacea

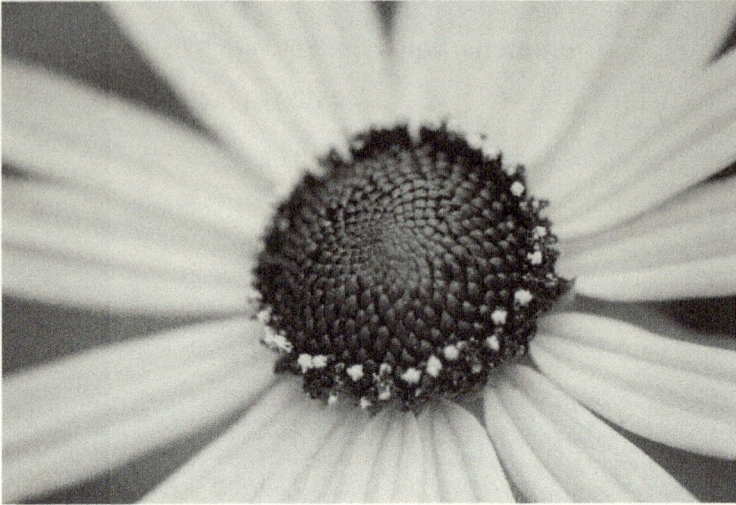

Echinacea is one of the oldest herbal remedies used in the world. It is known to promote immune system health and may provide direct antiviral support. This healing herb has long been popular among herbalists, and it is now the subject of current scientific research and clinical trials. Echinacea's flowering parts and roots have proven effective in alleviating the symptoms of common cold, viral bronchitis, and upper respiratory tract infection. This natural antiviral may provide a healthier and occasionally more effective alternative to pharmaceuticals.

TIP: Use Echinacea to cure various skin problems, such as simple herpes, acne, psoriasis, ulcers, boils, burns, wounds, eczema, and abscess. Try fresh or dried Echinacea root in a homemade decoction. Start with 2 handfuls of the root and 1 liter of water. Bring them to a boil; allow them cook until the volume is reduced by ¼. Let the decoction cool, then strain. Store in a bottle for use within 3-4 days; wash the skin with it up to 3 times a day.

Availability: From most good herbal remedy shops. (e.g. avogel.co.uk, iHerb.com, Amazon.com)

Antiviral Properties: Polysaccharides, glycoproteins, alkamides, volatile oils, and flavonoids. An immunostimulant that helps the body boost its immune system. Echinacea is *primarily used for viral bronchitis*.

Collection & Preparation: Can be taken as an herb juice, a tincture or an oil, a freeze-dried capsule, or a tablet. You can also make a tea by drying the roots out for 2 weeks and brewing it with 8 oz. of water.

Dosage: 500-1000 mg of Echinacea 3 times daily is recommended to treat common cold symptoms. Juice 6-9 mL daily for 7 days and 0.75-1.5 mL of tincture, gargled then swallowed 2-5 times daily for 7 days. The most recommended method of consuming it is to tincture it. Avoid using for longer than 3 weeks.

Possible Side Effects: Itchiness or a rash. High doses of Echinacea may cause nausea, dizziness, insomnia, or headaches.

Contraindications: Do not take if suffering with autoimmune disorders such as MS. Avoid use during pregnancy or if allergic to ragweed. Also check with doctor for possible interaction with other medicine, e.g. heart medication, antifungal, or anti-anxiety drugs.

Alternatives: N/A.

Other Uses: Influenza, Urinary Tract Infections, Vaginal Yeast Infections, Genital Herpes, Gum Disease, Acne, Psoriasis, Cold, Sinus Infections, Candidiasis, Asthma.

3. Astragalus Root

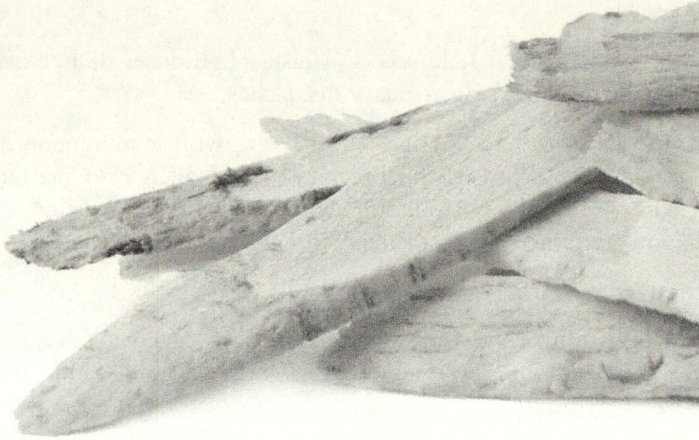

Astragalus is said to offer health benefits for a variety of conditions, including heart conditions. It appears to work by stimulating the immune system and has antioxidant properties that hinder the production of free radicals, which damage body cells and have been linked to health problems associated with aging.

Astragalus comes from the legume, or bean, family and multiple species exist. However, most herbal supplements will come from the *Astragalus membranaceus* plant. It is also known as *huang qi* or *milkvetch*.

TIP: Did you know that Astragalus acts as add-on to cancer therapies? It is a very useful complementary treatment during chemotherapy and reduces its side effects, such as fatigue, liver damage, lack of appetite. Additionally, it hinders cancer cell growth while accelerating a patient's recovery.

Availability: Most good herbal remedy stores. (e.g. iHerb.com, Amazon.com, naturesremedy.co.uk)

Antiviral Properties: Polysaccharides, choline, betaine, rumatakenin, [beta]-sitosterol. Astragalus has long been popular among other traditional Chinese treatments due to it's being an adaptogen, which means that it's great for helping the body against physical, mental, and emotional stress. It is *primarily used for colds and the Human Papillomavirus (HPV) infection, which causes warts.*

Collection & Preparation: It is available as a tablet, capsule, powder, or tincture. The root needs to be dried. Can also be made into a tea by mixing

3-6 oz. of dried root in 12 oz. of water.

Dosage: 200 mg of powder twice a day. Tea can be taken 3 times a day. Tincture can be taken 3 times a day – mix 10-15 drops of tincture in half glass of water.

Possible Side Effects: Can make your immune system more active, so will have an impact on those who suffer from an autoimmune disease.

Contraindications: Do not use if pregnant or breastfeeding, also avoid if you suffer from blood disorders.

Alternatives: N/A.

Other Uses: Dietary Supplements, Colds, Cancer, Arthritis, Asthma, HIV, AIDS, Energy Levels, Diarrhea.

4. Cat's Claw

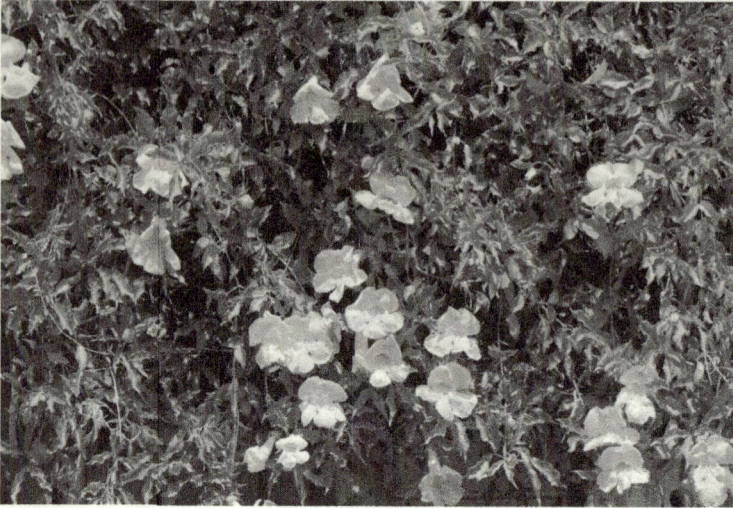

Cat's Claw is a Peruvian herb, *Uncaria tomentosa*, commonly called '*una de gato*' in Spanish. This "new" botanical nutrient has been studied at research facilities in Peru, Hungary, Austria, Italy, Germany, and England since the 1970s and continues drawing interest among the natural health care community. Some are even calling it the "Miracle Herb from the Rain Forest of Peru." Until now, it has been practically unheard of in the United States, but the benefits are clear. Studies have found that the herb can help with the treatment of stomach and intestine disorders, arthritis, menstrual irregularities, bursitis, depression, allergies, herpes, diabetes, cancer, lupus, and chronic fatigue syndrome.

TIP: Cat's Claw is great for treating candidiasis. Take Cat's Claw bark decoction and drink 2-3 times a day or have Cat's Claw capsules or extract.

Availability: Most good herbal remedy stores. (e.g. iHerb.com, Amazon.com)

Antiviral Properties: Quinovic acid glycosides, which work to protect the body's immune system. Cat's Claw is *primarily used for the herpes virus*.

Collection & Preparation: It is available as a tea by crushing the vines and mixing them with boiling water. It's also available as capsules, tablets, or a tincture.

Dosage: 60-100 mg of extract per day. 20-50 drops of tincture up to 3 times a day.

Possible Side Effects: Headaches, dizziness, and vomiting. Can cause diarrhea if taken in excess.

Contraindications: Do not take if you suffer from low blood pressure, leukemia, or autoimmune diseases. Also avoid taking during pregnancy or while breastfeeding.

Alternatives: N/A.

Other Uses: Digestive Problems, Bronchitis, Asthma, Cancer, Colitis, Anti-inflammatory and Antifungal Issues, Crohn's Disease.

5. Elderberry

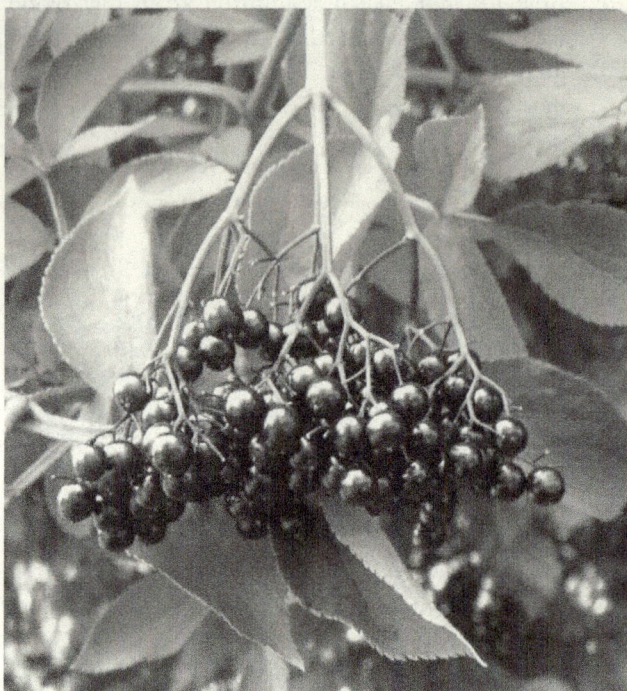

An extract of the common black elderberry, *Sambucus nigra*, can fight viruses by "disarming" the protein spikes on the particles' surface; these spikes help the virus penetrate host cells. Elderberry is popular for use in food and is considered one of nature's oldest remedies. According to some research, these therapeutic properties are attributed to flavonoids. It is these compounds that give Elderberry its color, which is where it derives its antioxidant and protective benefits. Elderberry is particularly effective against HIV and the herpes and influenza viruses. In lab tests, it was determined Elderberry could reduce infectivity of HIV strains and inhibit replication in four strains of the herpes simplex virus, and in a Norwegian independent study, it was determined the extract alleviated influenza symptoms.

TIP: Did you know that elderberries can be used to treat conjunctivitis? Use a decoction extracted from *Sambucus williamsii* flowers. Be sure to cool and strain the liquid extract before using it on your eyes.

Availability: In most good health food and herbal remedy stores. (e.g. iHerb.com, Amazon.com, lewtress.co.uk)

Antiviral Properties: Flavonoids – including quercetin, which coats viruses and prevents them from penetrating and infecting healthy cells. Elderberries are *primarily used against the influenza virus.*

Collection & Preparation: Can be taken as a juice or used in your food. You can also buy Elderberry liquid capsules or powder.

Dosage: Take the juice extracts for no longer than 12 weeks or 15mL 4 times a day. Do not let up on the dosage as Elderberry must stay consistently in the body for it to do its job.

Possible Side Effects: Nausea, vomiting, and severe diarrhea. Can also decrease blood sugar.

Contraindications: Do not use if you suffer from autoimmune diseases or take immune system suppressants. Do not take if you use a laxative.

Alternatives: N/A.

Other Uses: Reduces Cancer Cell Formation, Antioxidant, Protects Blood Vessels; Effective for Bleeding, Facial Neuralgia, Rheumatoid Arthritis.

Elderberries, raw
Sambucus spp.

Nutritional value per 100 g (3.5 oz)		
Energy	305 kJ (73 kcal)	
Carbohydrates	18.4 g	
Dietary fiber	7 g	
Fat	0.5 g	
Protein	0.66 g	
Vitamins	**Quantity**	**%DV**[†]
Vitamin A equiv.	30 µg	4%
Thiamine (B_1)	0.07 mg	6%
Riboflavin (B_2)	0.06 mg	5%
Niacin (B_3)	0.5 mg	3%
Pantothenic acid (B_5)	0.14 mg	3%
Vitamin B_6	0.23 mg	18%
Folate (B_9)	6 µg	2%
Vitamin C	36 mg	43%
Minerals	**Quantity**	**%DV**[†]
Calcium	38 mg	4%
Iron	1.6 mg	12%
Magnesium	5 mg	1%
Phosphorus	39 mg	6%
Potassium	280 mg	6%
Zinc	0.11 mg	1%
Other constituents	**Quantity**	
Water	79.80 g	

6. Lemon Balm

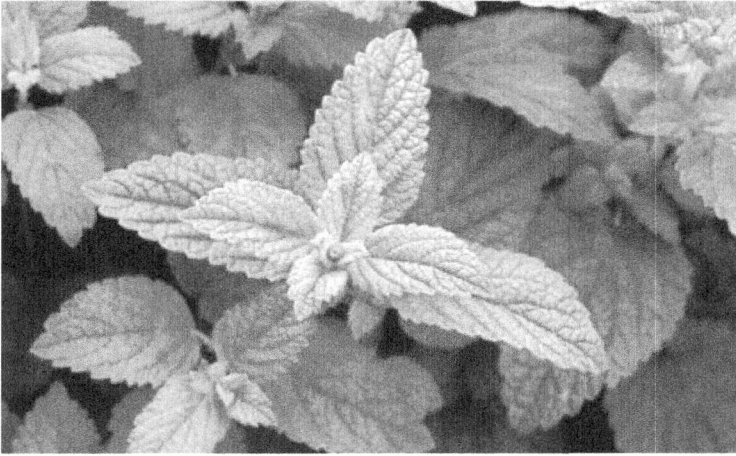

Lemon balm, known by its botanical name as *Melissa officinalis*, is applied for its calming properties. For centuries, lemon balm and its essential oils have been administered to alleviate indigestion, improve sleep, and ease anxiety and nervousness. This herb is a member of the mint family and has been found by experts to contain many great health properties. For instance, lemon balm was used by ancient Romans and Greeks in healing insect stings and bites.

Lemon balm is now naturalized to grow around the globe, but was native to south-central Europe. Often, it is planted in herb gardens because bees are attracted to it, but most insects are repelled by the tart aroma given off by the leaves – from which the essential oil citronella is extracted. The plant can grow up to 2 ft and shows light yellow flowers that blossom where the leaves and stem meet.

TIP: Lemon Balm counteracts dysmenorrhea, i.e. painful menses. Soak Lemon Balm leaves in water, then add the infusion to your bath water. Lemon Balm can also help start your menstruation cycle.

Availability: In most good herbal remedy and health food stores. (e.g. iHerb.com, Amazon.com, naturesremedy.co.uk)

Antiviral Properties: Terpenes, tannins, and eugenol, which have a strong calming and antiviral effect. Lemon Balm is *primarily used for the herpes virus.*

Collection & Preparation: Available as a capsule or can be made into a tea by mixing 1 oz. of fresh Lemon Balm leaves with boiling water. Also available as an essential oil or a tincture.

Dosage: 8-10 g of Lemon Balm leaves or 50-60 drops of tincture in water for no longer than 4 months. Can be taken as infusion of dried herb or fresh leaves (4-6 leaves). Drink twice a day.

Possible Side Effects: Abdominal pain, dizziness, wheezing, drowsiness.

Contraindications: Do not allow children under the age of 12 to take. Always consult a doctor before using it.

Alternatives: N/A.

Other Uses: Anxiety, Sleep Problems, Stomach Disorders, Anemia, Restlessness, High Blood Pressure, Insect Bites.

7. Licorice Root

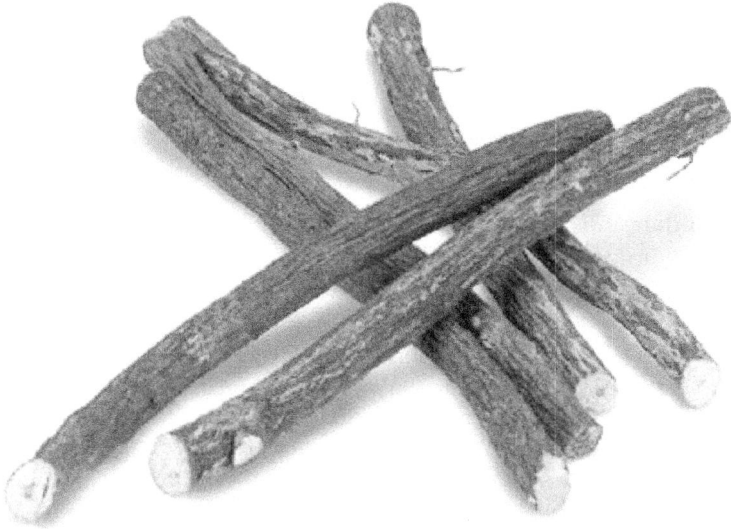

Licorice root has a long history of being used for medicinal purposes and flavoring or confectionery applications, especially among the Egyptians, Greeks, Chinese, and other Asian nations. It is called *gan cao* in Chinese and known as "sweet herb." The root has a distinct flavor, comprising a hint of anise, and tastes sweeter than sucrose (sugar). The underground stems and roots of this herbaceous perennial, *Glycyrrhiza glabra*, contains several healthy compounds: flavonoids, anethole, volatile oils, chalcones, plant sterols, asparagine, coumarins, and glycosides. Licorice root's use for flavoring in candies has recently been replaced by anise, but it's still a major ingredient in tobacco products, herbal lozenges, and natural medicines.

Some studies have suggested, though, that even with its health benefits, there is a key compound, glycyrrhizic acid, that can raise blood pressure levels if the root is used regularly and in large quantities. Applying processed licorice root is an alternative that lacks the acid. Look for deglycyrrhizinated licorice root (DGL root) instead.

TIP: Did you know that Licorice Root is a good concomitant with most herbs, and enhances their effectiveness, when taken in small doses? It is also known as a harmonizer and pacifier.

Availability: Most good herbal remedy and health food shops. (e.g. Amazon.com, hollandandbarrett.com)

Antiviral Properties: Flavonoids, volatile oils, plant sterols, coumarins, glycosides, asparagine, chalcones, glycyrrhizic acid, and anethole. Licorice

Root is *primarily used for viral hepatitis.*

Collection & Preparation: Can be prepared in food or bought in medicinal tincture form, powder, or capsules.

Dosage: 2 mL of powdered root in 1 cup of water (boil it and simmer for 10 minutes). Drink 3 times a day. Avoid using for more than 6 weeks.

Possible Side Effects: High blood pressure, low potassium levels, fatigue, water and sodium retention. Edema, dizziness, may reduce libido.

Contraindications: Do not use if you suffer from high blood pressure, diabetes, hormone sensitive conditions, kidney disease, hypertonia, or are pregnant or breast feeding.

Alternatives: St. John's Wort.

Other Uses: Cough, Bronchitis, Colitis, Lower Cholesterol, Ulcers, Skin Disorders, Liver Problems.

8. Olive Leaf

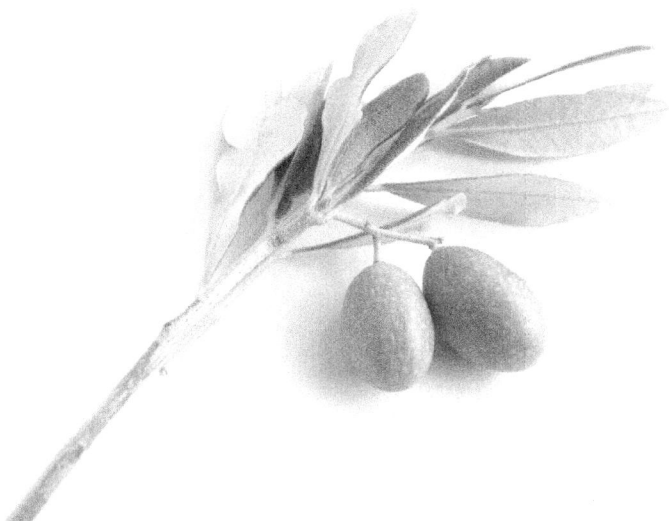

Olive trees and their leaves have long been popular for their ability to combat microbes and infections and provide protection for your skin, which is why extracts are applied as a powerful tonic to boost the immune system. Research conducted at the Rappaport Faculty of Medicine in Israel found that olive leaves virtually kill nearly all bacteria, especially E. coli and Candida albicans. After years of study, scientists isolated oleuropein as the specific molecule responsible for Olive Leaf's antibacterial properties.

TIP: Did you know that Olive Leaf is best used as an immunity booster? Oleuropein contained in olive leaves fights against viruses and bacteria that cause cold sores. Simply apply Olive Leaf extract over cold sores or take ¼ tsp. of Olive Leaf extract in a half-full glass of water.

Availability: Most good herbal remedy and health food shops. (e.g. iHerb.com, Amazon.com)

Antiviral Properties: *Olea europaea*, which blocks viral cell repetition and works to reduce fevers. Olive Leaf is *primarily used to fight the influenza virus.*

Collection & Preparation: Can be consumed with food (Olive oil) or purchased as a liquid extract.

Dosage: Liquid extract at 30 mL per day or 30-40 g with food.

Possible Side Effects: Can affect respiration allergies or cause allergic reactions if applying on skin.

Contraindications: Do not use if pregnant, breastfeeding, or suffering from diabetes.

Alternatives: N/A.

Other Uses: High Blood Pressure, Oral Herpes, Eczema, Measles, Insect Bites, Cancer, Age-related Diseases, Arthritis.

9. Black Seed

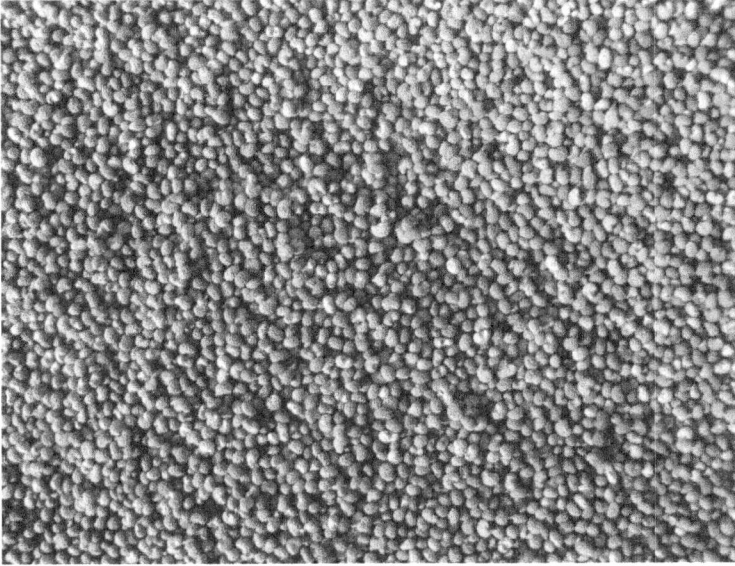

Even though it has gone by many names, such as black caraway, black cumin, black sesame, onion seed, and Roman coriander, *Nigella sativa* is primarily known today as black seed. The humble seeds of the annual flowering plant are immensely powerful – with the capability to heal a body poisoned by chemical weapons, destroy MRSA, and regenerate a diabetic's dying beta cells. Although too few know it exists, these tiny seeds have a long history of being used for their healing properties.

In fact, the earliest record of it being cultivated for use originates from ancient Egypt, nearly 3,300 years ago, where the extracted essential oil was discovered in the pharaoh Tutankhamun's tomb. Within the Arabic world, black cumin is called *Habbatul barakah*, which translates to "seed of blessing." Further, in Islam, it is taught that the prophet Mohammed called black cumin "a remedy for all diseases except death."

TIP: Did you know that Black Seed oil is used to treat common skin ailments? A decoction prepared from its seed and apple cider vinegar is applied over acne, rashes, psoriasis, eczema, dermatitis, allergies, wrinkles, burns, etc. It heals and nurtures the skin and makes it more beautiful.

Availability: In most good herbal remedy and health food shops. (e.g. iHerb.com, Amazon.com, amazingherbs.com)

Antiviral Properties: Thymoquinone, thymohydroquinone, dithymoquinone, thymol, carvacrol, nigellicine, and alpha-hederin – all of which work towards boosting your immune system. Black Seed is mostly known for its work in *HIV treatment*. It is also used for *pain relief*.

Collection & Preparation: Mix the oil with another liquid, such as juice or yogurt. The seeds must be heated. It is also available as a powder.

Dosage: 3 tsp. per day.

Possible Side Effects: Do not take if pregnant – Black Seed can prevent the uterus from contracting.

Contraindications: Do not take if you suffer from bleeding disorders, diabetes, or low blood pressure. Consult a doctor before consuming.

Alternatives: N/A.

Other Uses: Sore Throat, Headaches, Asthma, Hay Fever, Bronchitis, Constipation, Combating the Side Effects of Chemotherapy.

10. Green Tea

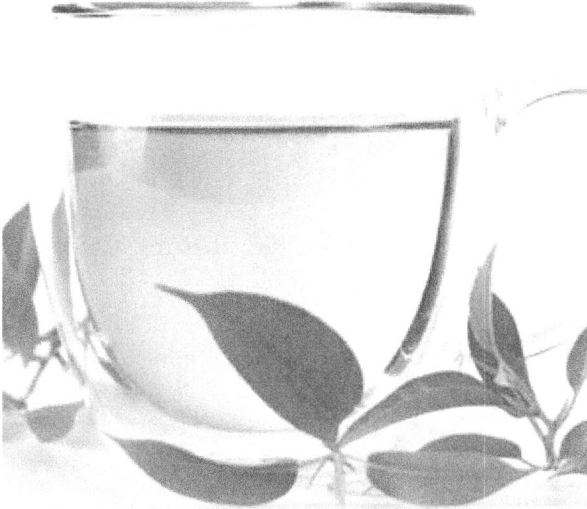

The health benefits of green tea, *Camellia sinensis*, were validated recently by scientific research, but this tea leaf has been used for more than 4,000 years as a natural remedy within traditional Chinese medicine. Flavonoids are at work in this herb, too. This group is called catechins, and they can inhibit infections, the influenza virus specifically, by binding to a certain protein, the haemagglutinin, and preventing entry into the living cells. Research conducted in China, studying isolated catechin derivatives and Green Tea extract, shows that the viral enzymes DNA polymerase and reverse transcriptase that support viral replication can be blocked. Tested compounds were determined to be effective in hindering the hepatitis B and herpes simplex viruses and HIV.

TIP: Did you know that Green Tea can help with hair problems, especially with male baldness? Drink 1 cup of Green Tea 3 times a day or purchase Green Tea capsules to take twice a day.

Availability: In most good health food and herbal remedy stores.

Antiviral Properties: Catechins, which inhibit viral infections by binding the haemagglutinin, preventing it from infecting healthy cells. Green Tea is *primarily used to prevent the influenza virus from spreading further.*

Collection & Preparation: Available as tea leaves or tea bags. Brew the tea by mixing 2 oz. of leaves with 6 oz. of water. Green Tea is also available as a capsule or tablet to be taken 3-4 times daily.

Dosage: No more than 3 cups a day.

Possible Side Effects: Headaches, nervousness, sleep problems, constipation, dizziness, and irritability.

Contraindications: Do not use if pregnant or breastfeeding or suffering from blood pressure issues. Do not exceed 2 cups a day if suffering from anxiety disorder or irregular heart rate.

Alternatives: N/A.

Other Uses: Cataracts, Dental Diseases, Rosacea, Cancer, Weight Loss, Cholesterol, Alzheimer's.

11. Ashwagandha (*Withania somnifera*)

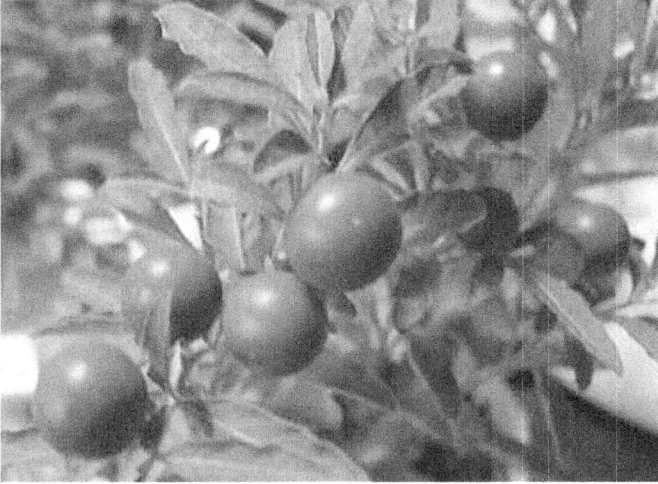

The ashwagandha plant, *Withania somnifera*, has a long history of use within Ayurvedic medicine. It has been used to relieve stress, enhance libido, and as a remedy for exhaustion and general weakness. An important aspect of Ayurvedic medicine are formulas referred to as Rasáyana tonics, and they are applied consistently over time to help regenerate body and brain tissues. Ashwagandha is one of the rare herbs that are so potent, offering numerous health benefits, that experts of Ayurveda consider it a Rasáyana therapy that can be applied on its own.

TIP: Did you know that Ashwagandha can heal carbuncles in as little as 4 weeks? Leaves can heal it at a much faster rate. Note that some people may face difficulty digesting Ashwagandha. They may want to take Ashwagandha with digestive herbs like Pepper and Ginger.

Availability: In most good herbal remedy stores. (e.g. iHerb.com, Amazon.com)

Antiviral Properties: Steroidal lactones and alkaloids, which work to rejuvenate the body and mind. Ashwagandha is *primarily used to fight viral infections and repair the body afterwards.*

Collection & Preparation: Ashwagandha can be taken in capsule or powder form. Boil 1 tsp. of powder with 1 cup of milk on low heat for 10 minutes, then blend with 1 tsp. of a natural sweetener, such as honey, and ¼ tsp. of a spice, such as ginger or cinnamon. Add ½ tsp. of ghee (clarified butter) to boost the herb's power.

Dosage: Initially, begin with smaller dose to see if it suits your body. Take

67

2 g twice a day for 1-3 months. It is advised to take a break of 1-2 weeks after consuming it for 2 straight months. For leaves in powder form, take 3-5 g; for root in powder form, take ¼ to ½ tbsp.

Possible Side Effects: Stomach upset, diarrhea and vomiting, drowsiness, low blood pressure, lower blood sugar, abdominal pain, shallow breathing.

Contraindications: Do not use if you suffer from diabetes, congestion, blood pressure issues, stomach ulcers, or autoimmune diseases. Avoid during pregnancy or while breastfeeding. Do not take Ashwagandha if you're allergic to it (if you're unable to digest tomatoes, potatoes, or peppers – you should avoid this herb). Ashwagandha may adversely affect the actions of some medications, hence you should consult your doctor before taking it.

Alternatives: Shatavari.

Other Uses: Alzheimer's, Anxiety, Fatigue, Stress, Lack of Concentration, Stabilizes Blood Sugar, Lower Cholesterol, Anemia, Cancer, Anorexia, Arthritis.

12. Ginseng

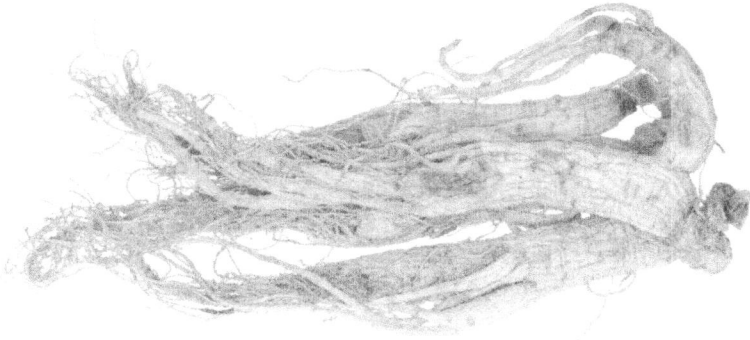

Traditional Chinese medicine has used *Panax ginseng* to improve digestion, strengthen the lungs, enhance energy, and calm a restless spirit. This herb is an adaptogen, which means it boosts the adrenal system to help heighten your body's resilience and promote system balance during stressful circumstances. It is a standard ingredient in dietary supplements, even energy drinks, that improve mental alertness, sports performance, and vitality. Additionally, Asian Ginseng contains anticancer and anti-inflammatory properties and has been shown to promote immunity, especially when fighting a cold or the flu. When attempting to purchase this herb, be aware that three different herbs are commonly known as 'ginseng': American ginseng (*Panax quinquefolius*), Asian or Korean ginseng (*Panax ginseng*), and Siberian ginseng (*Eleutherococcus senticosus*). Even though Siberian ginseng provides many of the same properties as American and Asian ginseng, it is not considered a "true" ginseng.

TIP: Did you know that Ginseng has the ability to balance the blood pressure? In case of hypotension, it increases the blood pressure, and at the same time it restores blood pressure to normal in case of increased blood pressure.

Availability: In most good herbal remedy stores. (e.g. iHerb.com, Amazon.com, simplysupplements.co.uk)

Antiviral Properties: Ginsenosides, which work in many areas of the body and help improve the body's resistance to stress and increases vitality. Ginseng is *primarily used to fight influenza.*

Collection & Preparation: Available as a capsule, powder, tincture, tablet or can be taken as a tea from fresh roots or dried root powder.

Dosage: Dry root – 1 g daily and don't take for longer than 3 months at a time. Then a break of 1 week to 3 months is recommended.

Possible Side Effects: Nervousness, insomnia, anxiety, hypertension, rise in blood sugar, edema, headaches, and stomach upset.

Contraindications: Do not take if you suffer from diabetes, autoimmune diseases, are on *Warfarin* or antidepressants, or experience an acute fever or sore throat. Avoid while pregnant or breastfeeding. Not recommended for children or if you plan surgery within 10 days or less. Always discuss with health practitioner before using it.

Alternatives: Rhodiola.

Other Uses: Stress, Fatigue, Increase Energy Levels, Anemia, Antiaging, Diabetes, Cold, Alzheimer's, Heart Diseases, High Cholesterol, Cancer, Fibromyalgia.

13. Ginkgo Biloba

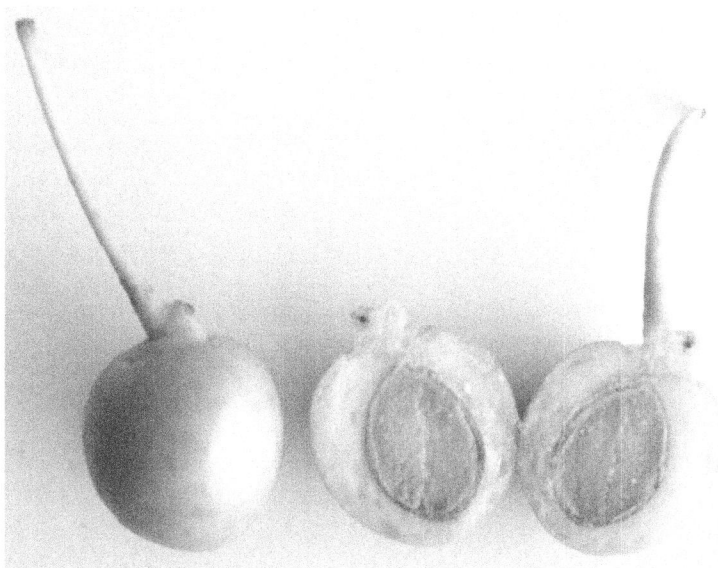

Ginkgo Biloba extract comes from the ancient herb, which has proven benefits for the elderly population, especially enhancing the body's use of oxygen, which then improves mental capabilities like concentration and memory function. Ginkgo has also been found to reverse retina damage and enhance long-distance vision. Scientific research has also confirmed its capability to treat depression, vertigo, tinnitus, sinusitis, and headache. Even though the Chinese have used ginkgo biloba, often called *Maidenhair*, medicinally for centuries – literally, Ginkgo trees have been traced back nearly 300 million years – modern applications are supported by German research, where the herb can be acquired with a prescription.

TIP: Ginkgo is a perfect remedy for aged people. It increases blood flow to the penis and ignites the sexual desire. Ginkgo also optimizes the flow of blood and enhances the sensation and consequently the pleasure. This way it promotes libido in both men and women. It also promotes lubrication and helps prevent ovarian cancer.

Availability: In most good herbal remedy stores. (e.g. iHerb.com, Amazon.com, woodshealth.com)

Antiviral Properties: Terpenoids and flavonoids, which improve blood circulation and kill bacteria. Ginkgo Biloba is *primarily used to fight the influenza virus*.

Collection & Preparation: Available in capsule, tincture, and tablet forms.

71

Dosage: 120-240 mg per day. The dosage depends on the illness you are trying to combat. It is recommended to reduce the dose after 10 days.

Possible Side Effects: Stomach upset, headache, dizziness, drowsiness, constipation, forceful heartbeat, high or low blood pressure, and allergic skin reactions.

Contraindications: Do not use if you suffer from diabetes, seizures, infertility, bleeding disorders, and avoid use for children. Avoid if pregnant or breast feeding.

Alternatives: Propolis.

Other Uses: Atherosclerosis, Dizziness, Tinnitus, Impotence, Dementia, Lyme Disease, Vertigo, Mood Disturbances, Alzheimer's, Asthma, Raynaud's Syndrome.

14. Colloidal Silver

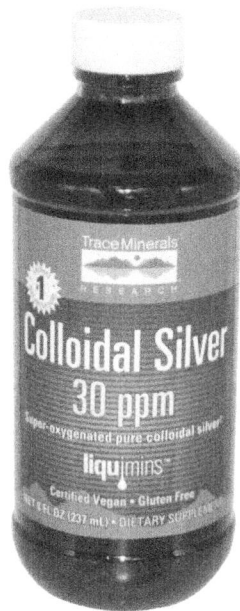

Colloidal Silver is a substance comprising silver particles being suspended in liquid, which is nearly impossible to filter or separate. Colloidal Silver and similar formulas that contained silver salts were popular with early 20th century physicians; however, in the 1940s, use was largely discontinued due to the discovery of safer, more effective modern antivirals and antibiotics. Only fifty years later, Colloidal Silver saw a resurgence in the market of alternative medicine, with claims that it has extensive "cure-all" properties. Colloidal Silver remains available in a variety of countries as a homeopathic remedy or dietary supplement.

TIP: Colloidal Silver is often used to treat skin ulcers. It reduces swelling and redness and prevents infection by helping wounds heal.

Availability: In most good herbal remedy stores. (e.g. iHerb.com, Amazon.com, highernature.com)

Antiviral Properties: Nanosilver has a toxicity to bacterial and viral pathogens. They prevent viruses from infecting healthy cells. Colloidal Silver is *primarily used to fight HIV*.

Collection & Preparation: Available as a spray, a tonic, drops or for use in a nebulizer.

Dosage: 1 oz. during a 24-hour period.

Possible Side Effects: If taken incorrectly, Colloidal Silver can impact on your internal organs and give your skin a blue-ish tint. It may also cause argyrosis or alter blood pressure.

Contraindications: Do not take when pregnant or breastfeeding.

Alternatives: N/A.

Other Uses: Ear Infections, Weight Loss, Gonorrhea, Arthritis, Bronchitis, Cancer, Ringworm, Psoriasis, Influenza.

15. Zinc

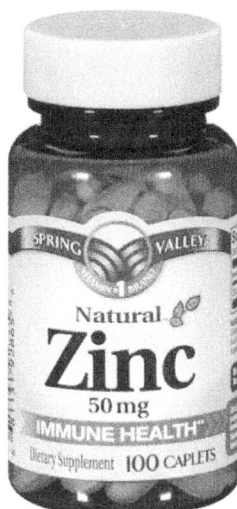

In a 2011 Cochrane review, researchers found that applying Zinc can be an effective element in treating colds. Doctors suggest taking Zinc supplements, in tablet, syrup, or lozenge form, within 24 hours of noticing the symptoms may enhance recovery and alleviate symptoms.

People with poor diet and digestive issues (like Crohn's disease); who are breastfeeding, strict vegetarians, or alcohol abusers are more likely to suffer a zinc deficiency and will benefit the most from Zinc supplements.

TIP: Avoid use of intranasal Zicam. These zinc-containing formulas have been withdrawn from the US market.

Availability: Available in most good herbal remedy stores. (e.g. iHerb.com, Amazon.com, myprotein.com)

Antiviral Properties: Pyrithione and hinokitiol. Zinc inhibits the rhinovirus replication making it *primarily used for the herpes simplex virus*.

Collection & Preparation: Available as a tablet, capsule, powder, or tincture.

Dosage: Do not take more than 11 mg for males and 8 mg for females per day.

Possible Side Effects: Coughing, stomach pain, fatigue.

Contraindications: Do not take if you suffer from diabetes, hemodialysis, arthritis or if you're pregnant or breastfeeding.

Alternatives: N/A.

Other Uses: Macular Degeneration, ADHD, Head Injuries, Weight Gain, Diarrhea, Stomach Ulcers.

16. Pau D'arco (Pink Trumpet Tree)

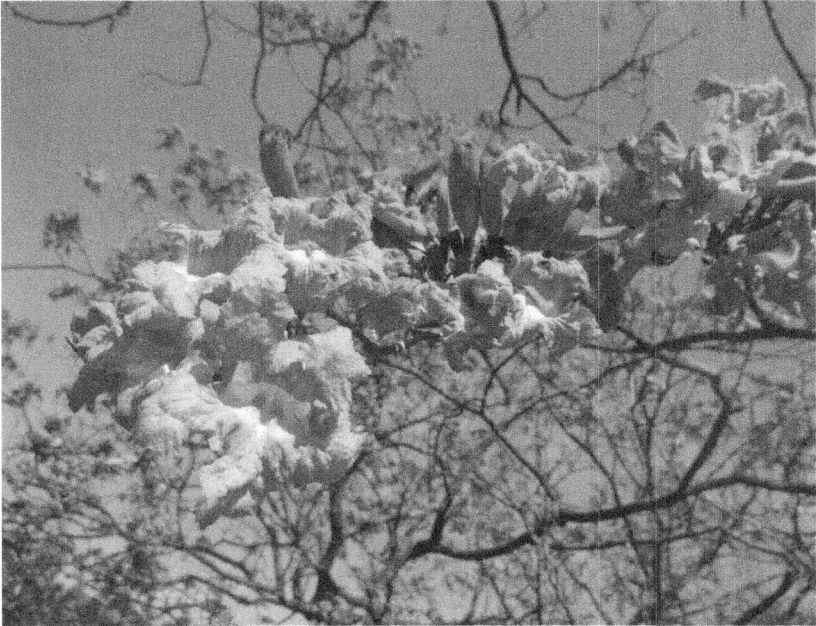

Pau d'arco, *Tabebuia avellanedae*, is native to South America and has been applied in herbal medicine to treat a variety of health issues, including ulcers and boils, general pain, various cancers, arthritis, dysentery, inflammation of the prostate gland, and fever. You may recognize the following names for pau d'arco: *Taheebo tree*, *Ipe roxo*, *Tabebuia avellanedae*, and *Lapacho*. There are reports of the medical use of this resilient tree from as early as 1873. The pau d'arco tree is known for its exceptionally hard wood; so much so, in fact, that its name means "bow stick" in Portuguese. This is because the tree is used to make hunting bows. Whereas, medicine is derived from the wood and bark.

TIP: Did you know that Pau D'arco has antibacterial and antifungal properties that help to cure a number of bacterial and fungal infections, e.g. candidiasis, athlete's foot, and even parasitic worms. To cure candidiasis, drink Pau D'arco tea, 2-3 cups a day, or take it as capsules or an extract.

Availability: In most good herbal remedy stores. (e.g. iHerb.com, Amazon.com)

Antiviral Properties: Naphthoquinones: lapachol and beta-lapachone. Pau D'arco is *primarily used for viral gastroenteritis and viral respiratory infections.*

Collection & Preparation: Available as tablets, capsules, a powder, a tincture, an extract, or a tea. The tea is made by boiling 1 tsp. of the powder in boiling water for 5-15 minutes.

Dosage: No more than 2 g per day.

Possible Side Effects: Nausea, diarrhea, vomiting, internal bleeding. If taken in high doses may cause high blood pressure, liver, and kidney damages.

Contraindications: Do not take if suffering from bleeding disorders or if you're pregnant or breast feeding. Stop use 15 days before scheduled surgery.

Alternatives: N/A.

Other Uses: Bronchitis, Stomach Inflammation, Anemia, Angina, Fever, Cancer, Candidiasis, Joint Pain, Boils, Wounds, Malaria, Gonorrhea, Syphilis.

17. St. John's Wort

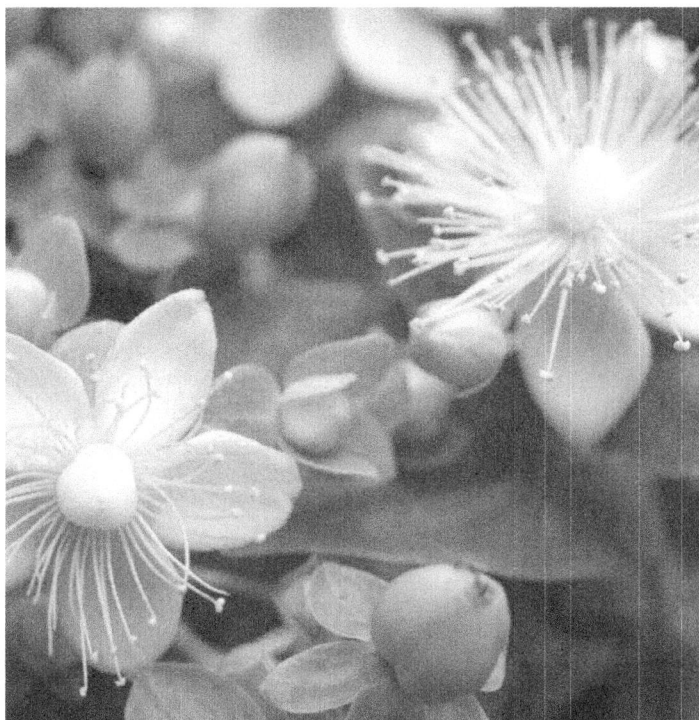

St. John's Wort, *Hypericum perforatum*, is a well-known herbal remedy that has also been called hypericum. The remedy is an extract of the plant's leaves and flowers. For several centuries, St. John's Wort has been used as a traditional medicine for healing mental health issues, especially depression, and wounds. This herbal remedy is still popular with the public because it's available for purchase at local shops and pharmacies, but it should be handled like a drug due to its pharmacologically active agents, such as hypericin. The specific element that gives St. John's Wort its healing properties isn't known, but it appears to have a direct effect on the enzymes and hormones noradrenaline, monoamine oxidase, and serotonin, its receptors, and its receptor expression.

TIP: St. John's Wort is good for punctured wounds, relieves post-operative pains and spasms after injury, or can be used instead of morphine after operation. Not only that, but it can also resolve problems related to children bedwetting.

Availability: In most good herbal remedy stores. (e.g. iHerb.com, Amazon.com)

Antiviral Properties: Naphthodianthrones (hypericin, pseudohypericin, protohypericin, protopseudohypericin, and cyclopseudohypericin), flavonoids (quercetin, rutin, and luteolin), hyperforin, several amino acids, and tannins. St. John's Wort is *primarily used for hepatitis B, herpes,* and *HIV.*

Collection & Preparation: Available as tablets, a liquid extract, a tincture, or a tea. The tea is made by mixing 1-2 tsp. of the herb with boiling water.

Dosage: The standard dosage is 300 mg 3 times a day.

Possible Side Effects: Dry mouth, sensitivity to sunlight, dizziness, stomach upset. If taken in high doses, can cause high blood pressure, skin rashes, diarrhea, insomnia, headache.

Contraindications: Do not take if you're using birth control pills, blood thinners, cancer drugs or you have high blood pressure, high cholesterol, bleeding disorders, or cataract. Also avoid it if you take antidepressants or have schizophrenia. Stop taking it at least 2 weeks before planned surgery.

Alternatives: Licorice Root.

Other Uses: Depression, Hydrophobia, Anxiety Disorders, Wounds and Injury to Nerves, Spasms After Injury, Insect or Snake Bites, Fibromyalgia.

18. Cordyceps (Caterpillar Fungus)

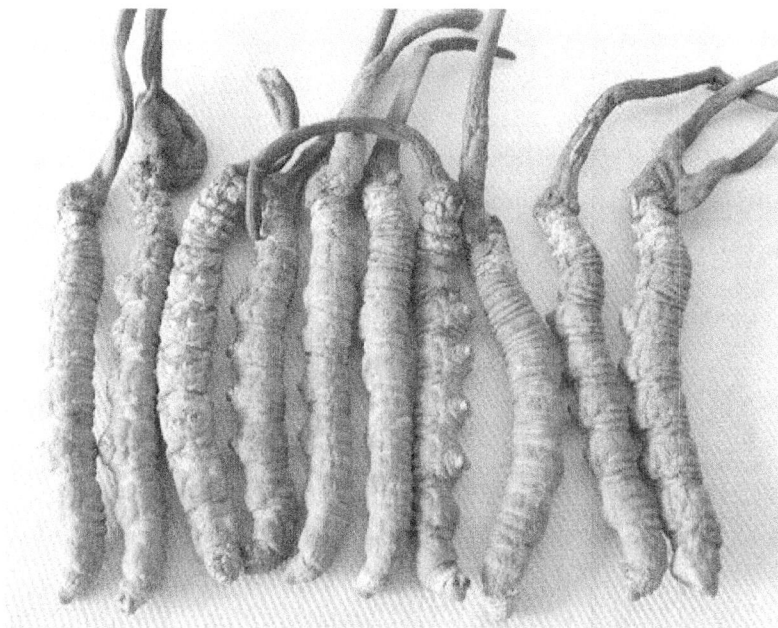

Cordyceps is a fungus that grows in the upper altitudes of the Himalayan mountains and the Tibetan plateau. Do not confuse this with your everyday, local grocer's mushroom. Technically, it is a caterpillar *and* a fungus. The fungus attaches directly to a caterpillar, then consumes the carcass as its food. Stems that grow from this combination produce spores seeking out hosts of their own. Cordyceps has been applied as an herbal medicine for numerous issues and as an aphrodisiac for centuries in China and Tibet. Despite its benefits, Cordyceps was so expensive its use was restricted to those with great wealth.

TIP: Did you know that Cordyceps has a great impact on the entire cardio-vascular system? It cures heart-related problems and enhances the circulation of the blood. Also regulates the blood pressure and strengthens the heart muscles, regulates its rhythm, and remarkably increases cardiac hypoxia tolerance.

Availability: In most good health food and herbal remedy stores. (e.g. gratefulgoose.com, iHerb.com, Amazon.com)

Antiviral Properties: Nucleosides, steroids, polysaccharides, proteins, essential amino acids. Cordyceps are *primarily used for the hepatitis B virus.*

Collection & Preparation: Available as a tablet, capsule, powder or to eat in food or take as tea and tincture.

Dosage: The standard dosage is 4-8 g daily.

Possible Side Effects: Sickness, stomach upset, dry mouth, nausea, diarrhea, headache, constipation.

Contraindications: Do not use if you suffer from autoimmune disorders, bleeding disorders, if you have fever, or if you're pregnant or breastfeeding. Also avoid it if you're allergic to mushrooms or any other type of fungus.

Alternatives: Other varieties of mushrooms.

Other Uses: Kidney Disorders, Fatigue, Infertility, Libido Loss, Impotence, Cancer, Anemia, Irregular Heartbeat, Weakness, Weight Loss, Bronchitis, Arthritis, Malaria, Yellow Fever.

19. Rhodiola

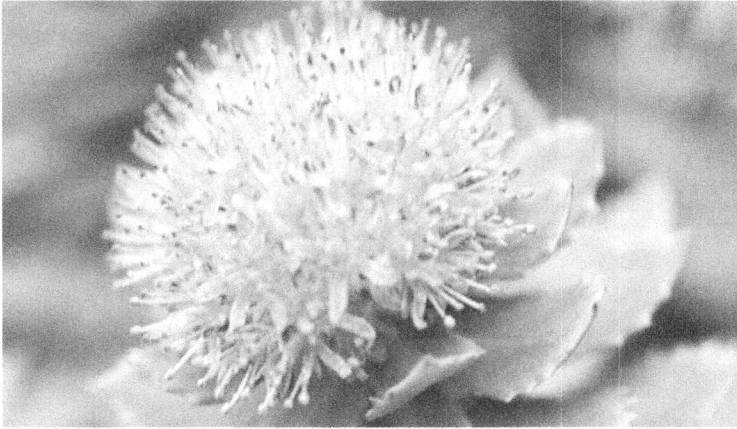

Rhodiola is a notable herb, long known for its strength as an adaptogen. For that property, it has a varied history of medicinal uses. Greek physician Dioscorides included *Rhodiola rosea* and its medicinal applications in the prominent medical text *De Materia Medica* in 77 AD. Chinese emperors sought out "the golden root" from Siberia, while the Vikings consumed Rhodiola to increase endurance and physical strength. It is noted that Mongolian doctors used it to treat cancer and tuberculosis, and the central Asian cultures brewed Rhodiola tea to alleviate cold and flu symptoms. To this day, it is applied to increase levels of energy, support the nervous system, enhance libido, fight depression, assist with weight loss, boost immunity, improve memory, and support capacity for exercise.

TIP: Did you know that Rhodiola relieves the symptoms of fatigue and enhances physical performance? It is known to regulate the hormones and improve muscular strength.

Availability: In most good herbal remedy stores. (e.g. pureclinica.com, iHerb.com, Amazon.com)

Antiviral Properties: Salidroside. Rhodiola is an adaptogen that works *primarily to combat stress in the body and fight off the common cold.*

Collection & Preparation: Available as a tablet, capsule, or tincture.

Dosage: No more than 600mg per day. Do not take for longer than 10 weeks at a time.

Possible Side Effects: Anxiety, restlessness, insomnia, nausea, confusion, irritability.

Contraindications: Do not take if you're pregnant or breastfeeding. Avoid using with stimulant drugs or if you suffer from bipolar depression with manic behavior.

Alternatives: N/A.

Other Uses: Increasing Energy, High Cholesterol, Hypoxia, Alzheimer's, Anxiety, Tuberculosis, Depression, Anemia, Cancer, Diabetes.

20. Boneset

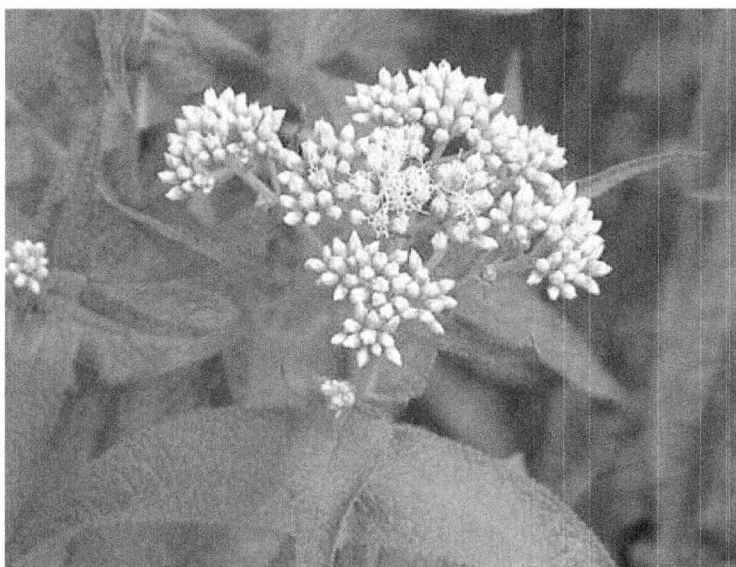

Boneset, *Eupatorium perfoliatum*, acquired its common name from its capacity to break the lethal fevers, so severe they were associated with being "bone deep" in a person's body, then called "bone fever," that developed with influenza. This herb has long been known as an effective treatment of influenza and fever; a prominent American herbalist, Dr. Edward E. Shook, was writing about boneset's prowess in World War I, when influenza took the lives of nearly 8 million people. Even earlier than that, Native Americans were using boneset to alleviate bodily aches and pains and enhance healing broken bones. Applying the herb as a tea or infusion did not become popular until much later, as many early applications of boneset took the form of topical plasters or poultices.

TIP: If you get constipated, take Boneset. It helps in proper bowel movement and gives relief. It can also improve digestion and is considered as a good appetizer.

Availability: In most good herbal remedy stores. (e.g. iHerb.com, Amazon.com)

Antiviral Properties: Calcium, magnesium, PABA, potassium, and Vitamins C and B-complex. Boneset is *primarily used to treat the influenza virus.*

Collection & Preparation: Available as a tincture, tablets, capsules, or a tea. The tea can be made by mixing 1 oz. of leaves with boiling water.

Dosage: The standard dosage is 2 g of leaves and flowers. It should not be taken for longer than 2 weeks' time.

Possible Side Effects: Liver damage, vomiting, stomach upset, weakness, diarrhea.

Contraindications: Do not take if you have an allergy to ragweed, if you suffer from liver or kidney disease, or if you're pregnant or breastfeeding.

Alternatives: N/A.

Other Uses: Joint Pain, Dengue, Anorexia, Fluid Retention, Increase Sweat and Urine Output, Anhidrosis, Digestive Problems, Malaria.

21. Eleuthero (Siberian Ginseng)

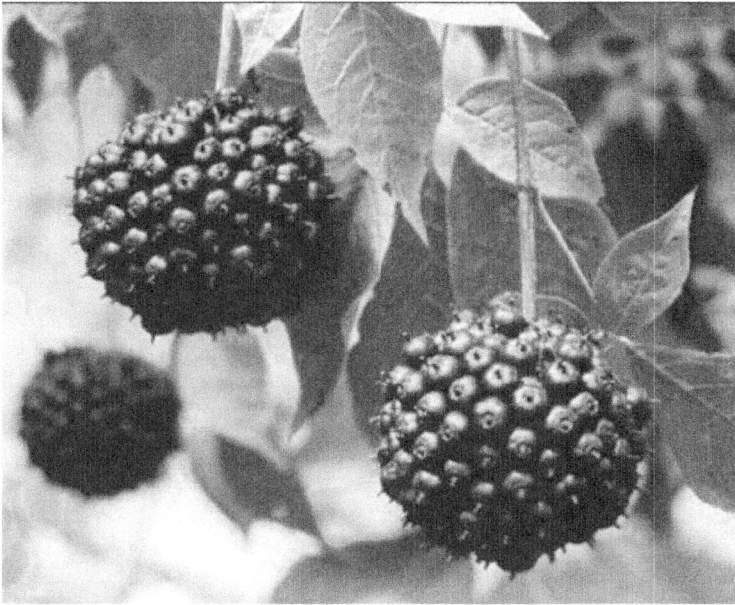

Eleuthero is also called Siberian ginseng, *Eleutherococcus senticosus*, and has been prized as an adaptogen for centuries in Russia, China, and other Eastern countries. As previously mentioned, it is not considered a "true" ginseng like the American and Asian ginsengs because of its unique active chemical components. These active components are called eleutherosides and are believed to support immunity. Traditionally, Siberian ginseng has been applied to enhance vitality, energy, and longevity, plus reinforce the immune system against cold and flu.

TIP: Siberian Ginseng is great to help overcome altitude sickness. It relieves this sickness by improving the supply of oxygen in the blood. You can take Siberian Ginseng in a capsule form (300 mg per day) or 10 drops of tincture in ¼ glass of water. Drink it twice a day.

Availability: In most good health food and herbal remedy stores. (e.g. naturesremedy.co.uk, iHerb.com, Amazon.com)

Antiviral Properties: Polysaccharides, which increase the body's production of interferon. Eleuthero is *primarily used for the herpes simplex virus*, but it also *works to boost the immune system, helping the body fight the cold and flu virus.*

Collection & Preparation: Available as a tablet, capsule, tincture, or an extract.

Dosage: 500 mg per day for viral infections. Be careful; if you have been applying Siberian Ginseng for more than 2 months, be sure to take break from the herb for 2-3 weeks.

Possible Side Effects: Drowsiness, depression, insomnia, headache, hypertension, anxiety, muscle spasms, changes in heart rate.

Contraindications: Do not take if you suffer from bleeding disorders, diabetes, prostate disorders, heart conditions, hormone sensitive conditions, high blood pressure, or mental conditions. Avoid if pregnant, menstruating, or breastfeeding.

Alternatives: Other Ginseng products.

Other Uses: High Blood Pressure, Kidney Disease, Stress, Fatigue, Cancer, Diabetes, Insomnia, Arthritis, Alzheimer's, Debility, Hyperthyroidism.

22. Redroot

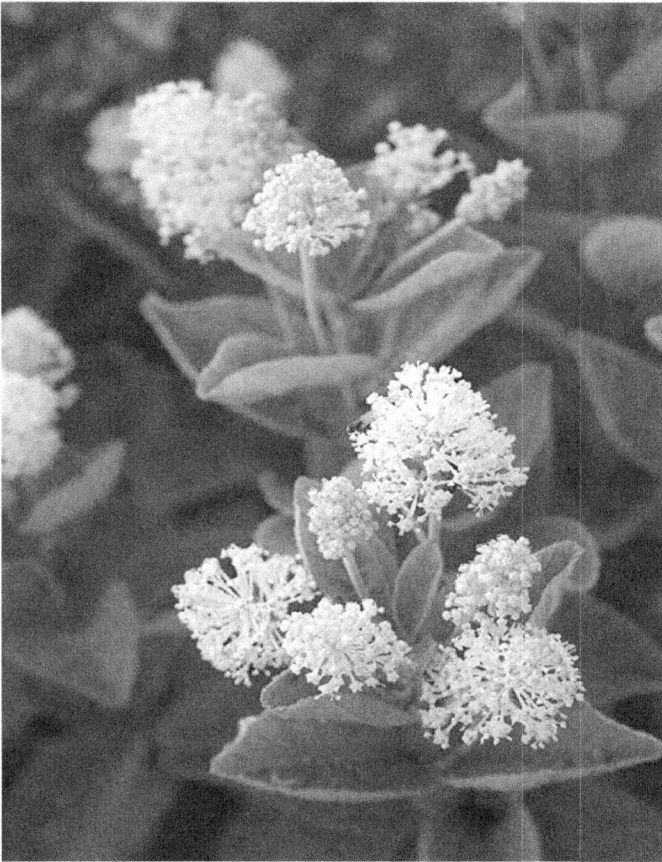

Redroot is an underutilized, yet powerful medicinal plant. Many Eclectic texts display little to no information on it, but Redroot received better representation in the *King's American Dispensatory* (1898 edition). Until then, due to little therapeutic evidence, the plant suffered under the misrepresentation of being virtually useless until the middle of the 20th century. That misrepresentation resulted from the leaves of the plant being used rather than the roots – which were far more powerful and provided different support. Additionally, Western medicine took so long to recognize the importance of the spleen and the lymphatic system in terms of treating disease and general function.

TIP: Redroot can be used for treating tonsillitis. Apply Redroot bark by boiling it in water for 15 minutes and gargling with the infusion at least 2 times a day.

Availability: In most good health food and herbal remedy stores. (e.g. gratefulgoose.com, iHerb.com, Amazon.com)

Antiviral Properties: Tannins, triterpenes, flavonoids, and ceanothine. Redroot is *primarily used for the treatment of asthma, bronchitis, and coughs.*

Collection & Preparation: Available as a tincture or a capsule. Redroot can also be made into a tea by adding the dried root powder to boiling water for 10-15 minutes.

Dosage: 1 tsp. 3-4 times a day.

Possible Side Effects: Headache, dizziness, insomnia, irregular heartbeats, vomiting, diarrhea, and loss of appetite.

Contraindications: Do not take if you're using iron supplements, blood thinners, if you are pregnant or breast feeding.

Alternatives: Ceanothus ovalis.

Other Uses: Dental Care, Fever, Gonorrhea, Blood Impurity, Spleen Diseases, Insomnia, Dysentery, Skin Diseases.

23. Reishi Mushroom (Ganoderma)

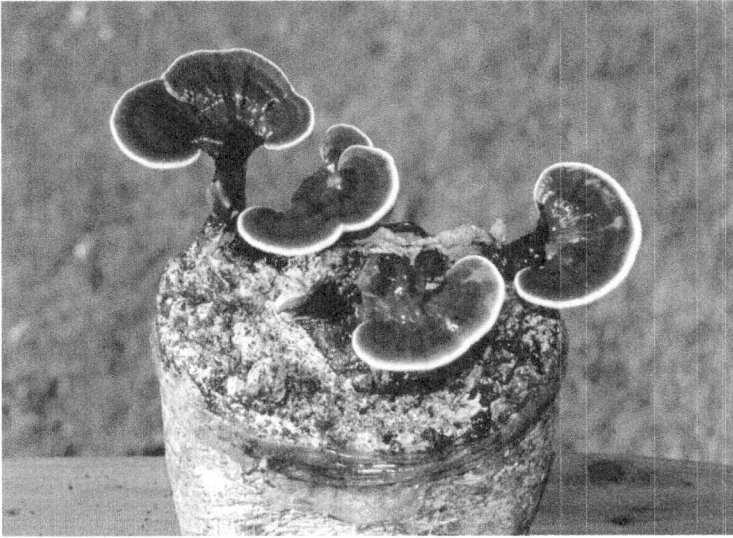

Red reishi mushroom contains beta-glutens, the water-soluble polysaccharides, and hetero-beta-glucans and is considered the highest quality among the mushrooms available. Those polysaccharides are known to lower blood pressure, enhance the immune system, and fight tumors. One of the other red reishi active ingredients is the ling zhi-8 protein, which supports immune system function, as well. Medical patients going through an organ transplant or taking immunosuppressive medicines need to practice caution when taking red reishi supplements. It is considered very safe, but an immune-modulating substance could produce an adverse interaction.

TIP: Did you know that Reishi Mushroom is very well known as an anti-cancer treatment? It reduces anabolic activity, hence making it anti-tumor and helps the healing process. It also rids the body from toxins, strengthens the immune system, detoxifies the liver, protects the good cells from radiation. Therefore, to better protect the patient from radiation, it is advised that the administration of Reishi should start before radiation therapy and continue after exposure. It is a very important supplement for the treatment of liver cancer.

Availability: In most good health food and herbal remedy stores. (e.g. iHerb.com, Amazon.com)

Antiviral Properties: Polysaccharide, which helps protect damaged cells. Reishi Mushrooms are *primarily used to fight viral gastroenteritis, laryngitis,* and *Epstein Barr virus.*

Collection & Preparation: Available as an extract or to be used in food.

Dosage: Use 2-6 g per day of raw Reishi Mushrooms or a similar dosage of the concentrated extract would also work. For best results, take Reishi Mushroom on an empty stomach in the morning. Drink more water with Reishi Mushroom.

Possible Side Effects: Dryness of the mouth, throat, and nasal area along with itchiness, stomach upset, nosebleed, bloody stools, blood pressure fluctuations, breathing problems.

Contraindications: Do not take if you're suffering from bleeding disorders, low blood pressure, thrombocytopenia or if you are pregnant or breastfeeding. Also avoid for children up to 12 years.

Alternatives: Other mushroom products.

Other Uses: High Cholesterol, Kidney Disease, Cancer, Aging, Autoimmune Diseases, Fatigue, High Blood Pressure, Alzheimer's, Atherosclerosis, Chest Pain, Chronic Hepatitis B, Anemia.

24. Turmeric

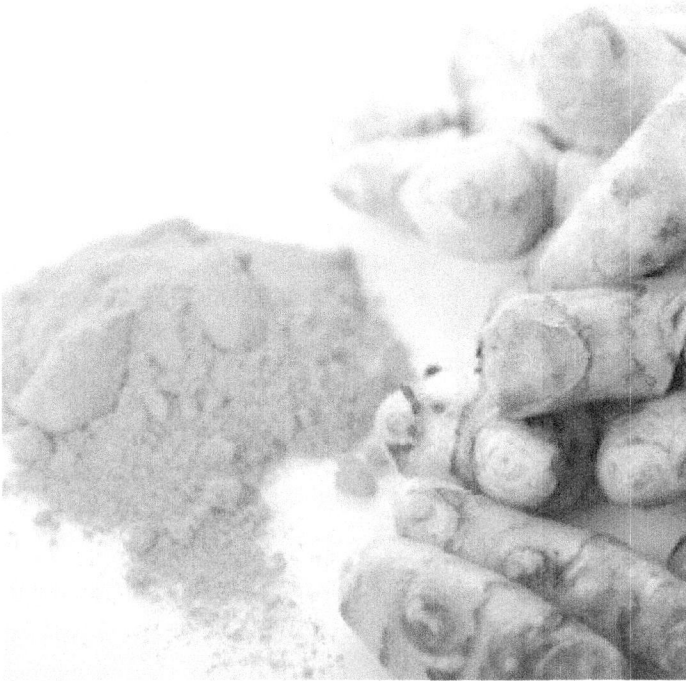

Turmeric comes from a tropical plant, which is a member of the ginger family. The root stalk of this plant has a long history of being used in Chinese and Indian Ayurvedic medicine to treat conditions such as depression, heartburn, fibromyalgia, diarrhea, colds, and stomach bloating. Curcumin is one of Turmeric's main components and is said to provide healing properties.

TIP: If you think you are unwell, no matter how seriously, and your disease has not been diagnosed, take Turmeric for a month! Because Turmeric does not mix with water and it's not fully ingested by the small intestine mucosa, try mixing Turmeric with a little black pepper to make the absorption more effective. It will increase the absorption considerably. You can also add sesame, olive, or coconut oil to dissolve it.

Availability: In most good health food and herbal remedy stores. (e.g. iHerb.com, Amazon.com)

Antiviral Properties: Curcumin, which interferes with the reproduction of viral cells. Turmeric is *primarily used for the liver problems virus, Crohn's disease,* and *HIV*.

Collection & Preparation: Available as tablets, a powder, a tincture, a juice, an oil, or a spice to use with food.

Dosage: Turmeric root can be taken orally every day in divided doses. A standard dosage consists of 1.5-3 g. To consume in a tea, steep 1-1.5 g of dried root in 150 mL of water for 15 minutes; drink twice a day. Do not exceed 8 g of Turmeric per day.

Possible Side Effects: Stomach upset, nausea, altered heartbeat, risk of bleeding, dizziness, or diarrhea. May cause allergies like psoriasis or dermatitis.

Contraindications: Do not take if you suffer from gallbladder problems, obstruction of biliary tract, kidney stones, bleeding disorders, gastroesophageal reflux disease, hormone sensitive conditions, infertility, or iron deficiency. Avoid during pregnancy or if trying to conceive. Also avoid its use 15 days before planned surgery. Consult your doctor in case of diabetes or breast cancer. Simultaneous use with Clove reduces the desired actions of Turmeric.

Alternatives: N/A.

Other Uses: Arthritis, Heartburn, Cancer, High Cholesterol, Allergy, Anorexia, Liver Problems, Headaches, Ringworm, Skin Conditions, Prostatitis, Cuts and Wounds, Asthma, Slipped Disc, Anemia, Arthritis, Menstrual Cramps.

25. Rosemary

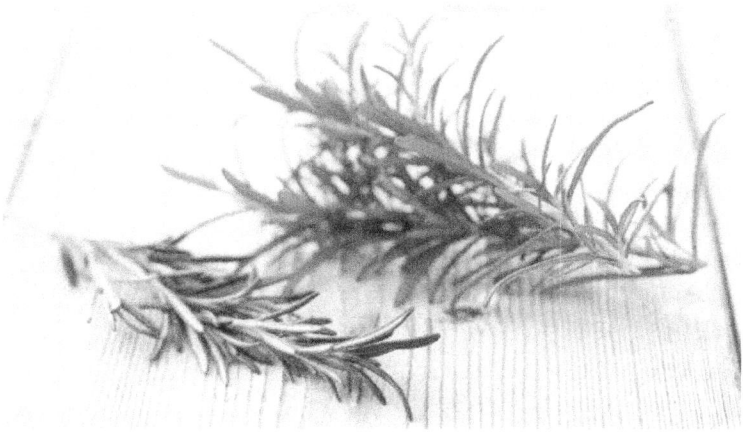

Lab testing has shown that Rosemary, *Rosmarinus officinalis*, has antioxidant properties. Antioxidants work to neutralize the harmful particles in your body called free radicals, which have a direct effect on DNA, weaken cell membranes, and even kill cells. In additional lab testing, Rosemary oil may have antimicrobial properties; it was able to destroy some fungi and bacteria inside test tubes. However, it wasn't clear that Rosemary would produce the same result in humans. Medicinally, Rosemary has been employed to support the nervous and circulatory systems, promote hair growth, enhance memory, and relieve muscle pain. One lab test determined that long-term, daily use could prevent thrombosis. Though none of the following uses have been confirmed with scientific review, Rosemary is also associated with alleviating indigestion, causing miscarriage (abortifacient), and increasing urine and menstrual flow. Rosemary is commonly added to food as a spice, especially in Mediterranean cooking, and as a fragrance in soaps and various cosmetics.

TIP: Did you know that Rosemary is proven to be effective for treating baldness? It is also effective in easing headache symptoms. Regular head and forehead massage with Rosemary oil is quite effective to get rid of headache.

Availability: In most good health food and herbal remedy stores. (e.g. iHerb.com, Amazon.com)

Antiviral Properties: Carnosic acid and rosmarinic acid, which boost the body's immune system and help fight off viral infections. Rosemary is *primarily used to fight bronchitis or asthma.*

Collection & Preparation: Available as an oil, a tincture, or a leaf that can be used in food or to make a tea. The tea is made by mixing fresh or dried leaves with boiling water for 10-15 minutes.

Dosage: The leaf standard dosage is 4-6 g per day. The oil is recommended at 0.1-1 mL dosage. Rosemary essential oil should not be taken by mouth. *For aromatherapy* – use 3-4 drops of essential oils for diffusing.

Possible Side Effects: Vomiting, uterine bleeding, kidney discomfort, skin sensitivity, increased risk of bleeding, increase or decrease in blood sugar levels.

Contraindications: Do not take if you have an allergy to aspirin; suffer from bleeding disorders, high blood pressure, ulcers, colitis; or if you're pregnant, breastfeeding, or trying to conceive.

Alternatives: N/A.

Other Uses: Digestive Problems, Alzheimer's, Skin Diseases, Cancer, Stress, Anxiety, Liver Disorders, Headache, ADHD, Amnesia, Gallbladder Complaints, Baldness.

26. Peppermint

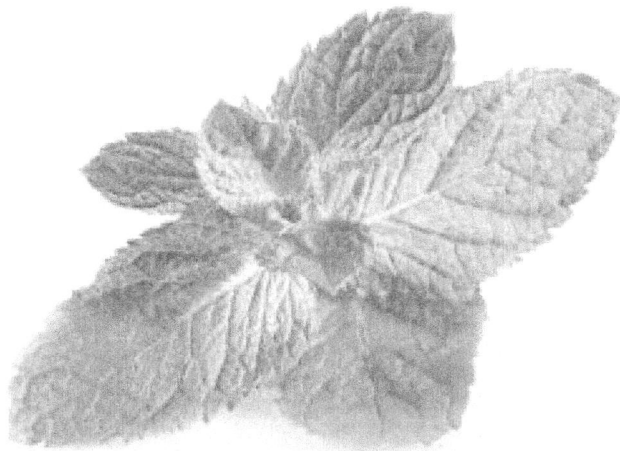

Peppermint, *Mentha piperita*, is a perennial plant with a popular flavor, used in products like tea, toothpaste, and gum, and healing properties. Scientific studies have shown that this herb can be used to ease indigestion, diarrhea, nausea, flatulence, or irritable bowel syndrome. Not only does it have a direct effect on your stomach, but it can provide a numbing or calming sensation. So, peppermint has also been used to alleviate cold and flu symptoms, menstrual cramps, headaches, anxiety and depression, and skin irritations. Under scientific review, peppermint has destroyed viruses, fungus, and specific types of bacteria in the test tube, which suggests it could contain antiviral, antifungal, or antibacterial properties.

TIP: You can ease your hangover with the help of Peppermint. It is known to soothe the irritated lining of the stomach and reduce the effects of hangover like nausea and vomiting due to intake of alcohol. Boil 10-12 Peppermint leaves in 1.5 cup of water for 5-10 minutes. Strain and drink tea 2-3 times a day. You can also have few drops of Peppermint essential oil in a glass of water.

Availability: In most good health food and herbal remedy stores. (e.g. iHerb.com, Amazon.com)

Antiviral Properties: Tannins and polyphenols, which work to fight off viral infections. Peppermint is *primarily used for treating chickenpox and similar viral conditions.*

Collection & Preparation: Available as tablets, capsules, a tincture, an oil, or as a tea. The tea can be made by blending the leaves with hot water for 5 minutes.

Dosage: *For digestion disorders* – 0.2-0.4 mL of Peppermint oil diluted in water or 2-4 g of dried herb extract 3 times daily. Do not swallow pure Peppermint leaves.

Possible Side Effects: Heartburn, flushing, headaches, mouth sores, lower blood sugar levels.

Contraindications: Do not take if you're suffering from diarrhea, gallbladder disease, or achlorhydria. Avoid during pregnancy or while breastfeeding.

Alternatives: Other plants in the mint family such as lemon balm.

Other Uses: Sinus Infections, Headache, Migraine, Sinusitis, Neuralgia, Hangover, Flu, Acidosis, Bloating, Heartburn, Nausea, Pain, Menstrual Problems, Stomach Problems.

27. Coriander

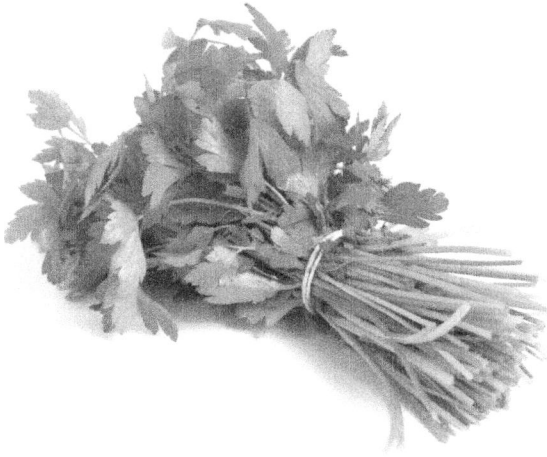

Coriander, *Coriandum sativum*, is a small, pleasantly aromatic, and spicy, hollow-stemmed plant found in the Apiaceae, or parsley, family. The herb's essential oil is extracted from the seeds, which measure a diameter of approximately 4-6 mm. Coriander has been used in traditional medicines and to flavor dishes since the ancient times. Though native to Southeastern Europe, coriander is grown across Europe, in the Middle East, Turkey, India, and China. In the West, coriander is often referred to as cilantro. This annual plant can reach 2 ft in height and displays branching stems, producing soft, smooth, deep green, leaves that may have two or three lobes. On a mature plant, small, light pink flowers will bloom that eventually turn into the oval-shaped, or globular, seeds (fruits).

TIP: Did you know that Coriander is very effective as a supplement treatment for heavy metal poisoning? Eat 1 cup of fresh Coriander leaves or chutney for 7 days every 6 months.

Availability: In most good health food and herbal remedy stores. (e.g. gratefulgoose.com, iHerb.com, Amazon.com)

Antiviral Properties: Monoterpenes, which fight viral cells. Coriander is *primarily used for assistance with the common cold or chickenpox.*

Collection & Preparation: Available as a tincture, an oil, a seasoning in food, or an infusion. The infusion can be made by mixing 150 mL of boiling water with powdered Coriander.

Dosage: The infusion can be taken before meals. The recommended dosage for the tincture is 10-20 drops.

Possible Side Effects: Increased sensitivity to sunlight, diarrhea, stomach pain, darkened skin, depression, lapse of menstruation, and dehydration. Excess intake may cause infertility.

Contraindications: Do not take if you suffer from diabetes, low blood pressure, or if you are allergic to mugwort, aniseed, caraway, fennel, or dill. Avoid if pregnant or breastfeeding.

Alternatives: N/A.

Other Uses: Upset Stomach, Flatulence, Heavy Metal Poisoning, High Cholesterol, Asthma, Hemorrhoids, Toothaches, Joint Pain, Bowel Spasms, Skin Diseases, Conjunctivitis, Painful Menses.

28. Sarsaparilla

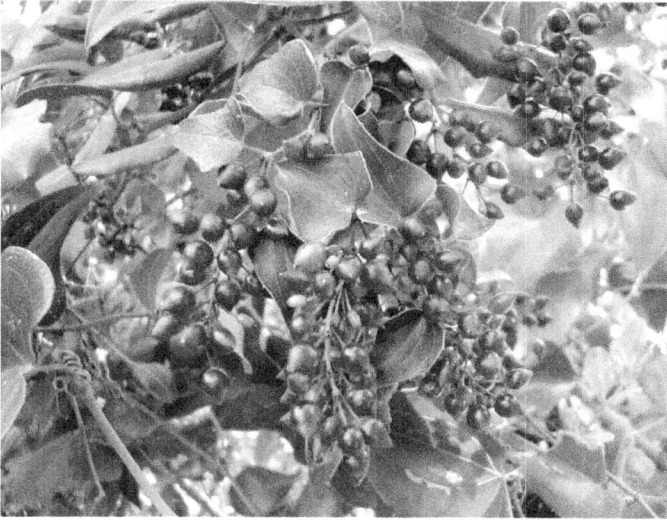

Sarsaparilla is the name of a perennial, trailing vine, berry-producing plant, and natural herb that is typically used in the treatment of psoriasis, eczema, and other skin disorders, but has also been applied in the treatment of syphilis, rheumatism, and liver disease. Promoted as a blood purifier, sarsaparilla products were used as sweat inducers, diuretics, tonics, and ingredients in several other applications, such as patent medicines. Sarsaparilla has also been employed to rejuvenate the male sex drive and in natural body-building compounds as an anabolic steroid replacement because testosterone is believed to be one of its main elements. Sarsaparilla is a native plant to Latin America, South America, Mexico, and the Caribbean islands, and it was exported to Europe in the 15th century.

TIP: Sarsaparilla is best known as a treatment for skin diseases. Grind its root with water. Apply on affected areas twice a day (works well for psoriasis).

Availability: In most good herbal remedy stores. (e.g. iHerb.com, Amazon.com)

Antiviral Properties: Sarsasapogenin, sitosterol, stigmasterol, pollinastanol, and flavonoids. Sarsaparilla is *primarily used to treat hepatitis B or HIV*.

Collection & Preparation: Available as capsules, a tincture, an extract, or a tea. The tea is made by mixing 1-2 tsp. of the powdered root into boiling water.

Dosage: No more than 2 g per day.

Possible Side Effects: Stomach irritation, occupational asthma.

Contraindications: Do not take if you suffer from asthma, kidney disease or if you're pregnant or breastfeeding.

Alternatives: N/A.

Other Uses: Syphilis, Rheumatoid Arthritis, Dysuria, Cancer, Diabetes, Leukemia, Skin Conditions, Gonorrhea, Digestive Disorders, Tick Bite.

29. Flaxseed

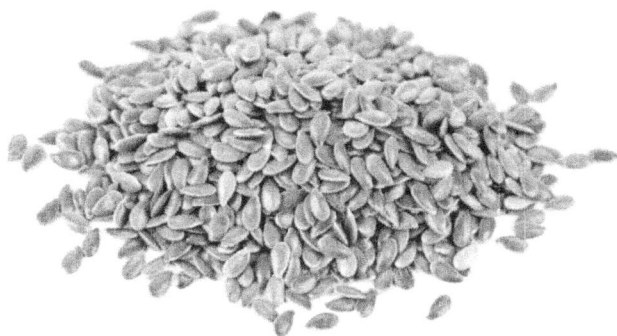

Flaxseeds are probably best known for their heart-health properties, from providing high fiber content to being a rich source (at 50-60%) of omega-3 fatty acids, specifically alpha linolenic acid. Potassium, protein, dietary fiber, B vitamins, antioxidants, and lignans (a group of phytoestrogens) can also be found in these powerful little seeds. While the seeds of the flax plant could be used whole, ground into a meal, or distilled to create Flaxseed oil (a vegetable oil also known as linseed), it is the seeds that are better for reducing the bad LDL cholesterol according to the *American Journal of Clinical Nutrition*. The *Journal of Clinical Oncology* determined that ground flaxseeds can hinder the growth of a prostate cancer tumor.

TIP: Flaxseeds are an excellent remedy if you have constipation. Simply take 1 tbsp. of bulk seed with a glass of water to avoid constipation.

Availability: In most good health food and herbal remedy stores. (e.g simplysupplements.co.uk, iHerb.com, Amazon.com)

Antiviral Properties: Lignans, which protect healthy cells from viral infections. Flaxseed oil is *primarily used for upper respiratory tract infections*.

Collection & Preparation: Available as an oil, a powder, capsules, or as seeds to eat.

Dosage: The standard dosage is 40-50 g per day of whole Flaxseeds. Generally, 1 tbsp. of Flaxseed may be mixed with 6-12 oz. of water or juice and taken up to 3 times daily.

Possible Side Effects: Bloating, gas, abdominal pain, constipation, heartburn, diarrhea, nausea, or may lower blood sugar levels when taken in large doses without water.

Contraindications: Do not take if you're suffering from bleeding disorders, diabetes, hormone sensitive conditions, hypertriglyceridemia, or blood pressure issues.

Alternatives: Other seed products.

Other Uses: Coronary Heart Disease, Constipation, Asthma, Blemishes, Cold, Alzheimer's, Colon Damage, Bladder Infections, Arthritis, Depression.

30. Basil

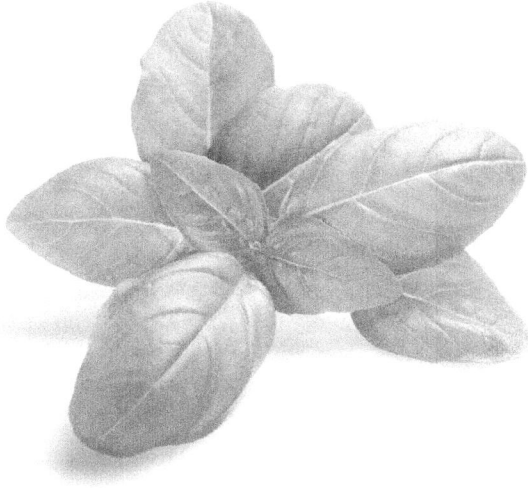

Basil, a bushy, annual plant, is among the oldest and most popular herbs, grown especially for its medicinal leaves and seeds, brimming with phytonutrients that have notable health benefits. In many traditions across the globe, this plant is considered a "holy herb."

Basil, *Ocimum basilicum*, belongs to the family Lamiaceae and is native to India, Iran, and tropical regions within Asia. This herb grows best in tropical climates. A mature plant can reach about 100 cm, on average, in height. Basil leaves are silky, light green, about 2.5 in long, 1 in broad, displaying in an opposite arrangement. The purple or white flowers can get quite large and appear in terminal spikes.

There are four varieties of Basil: Sweet basil, or "Mediterranean" cultivar, typically has light green leaves; Asian basil, *Ocimum sanctum*, has a stronger 'clove' flavor and displays large, hairy stems, pink flowers, and red or purple leaves; lemon basil has a "lemon" flavor; and Thai basil, *O. basilicum* or '*Horapha*,' shares characteristics with Asian basil but has a licorice-type aroma and displays narrow and pointed, light-green leaves.

TIP: Did you know that the seeds of Basil have a special medicinal effect on the body? They cool the body down, especially in the summer. So it's recommended to take Basil leaves in winter and Basil seeds in summer.

Availability: In most good health food and herbal remedy stores. (e.g. iHerb.com, Amazon.com)

Antiviral Properties: Ursolic acid, which coats viral cells. Basil is *primarily* *used for viral hepatitis.*

Collection & Preparation: Available as an oil, an essential oil, a powder or can be used as an herb in food or a tea.

Dosage: 500 mg of the leaf extract taken twice daily recommended for neurological or adaptogenic effects. Fresh Basil may carry pathogens and should always be washed before use. It's recommended to be used up to 6-8 weeks at a time.

Possible Side Effects: Low blood pressure, allergic skin reactions, diarrhea, increased risk of bleeding.

Contraindications: Do not take if you suffer from bleeding disorders. Avoid during pregnancy or while breastfeeding. Avoid taking Basil at least 2 weeks before planned surgery.

Alternatives: Other similar herbs, such as thyme.

Other Uses: Hair Loss, Fever, Repeated Miscarriage, Stress, Herpes Virus, Headache, Earache, Depression, Heat Stroke, Acid Reflux, Fluid Retention, Kidney Conditions, Mouth Infections, Tuberculosis, Malaria, Diabetes, Warts, Worm Infections.

31. Wood Betony

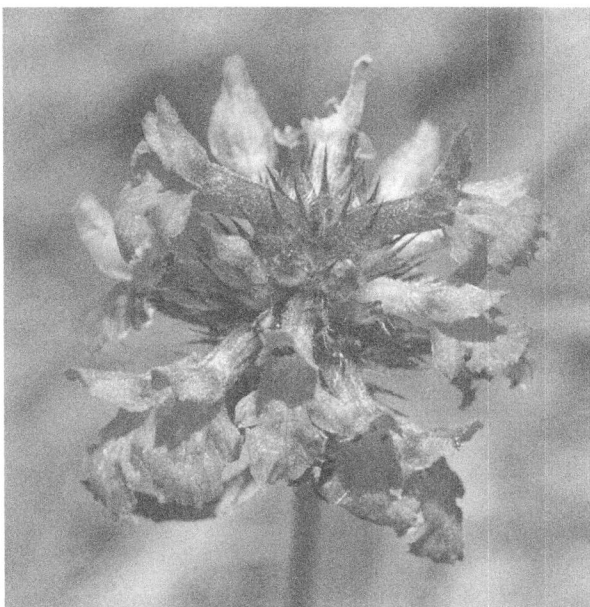

Wood Betony is a healing herb for many ailments. This perennial herb belongs to the family Labiatae and is known for being tall. It can grow up to 70 cm tall and contains numerous bright purple flowers, which grow in clusters of up to 15 on the very end of the upright, thick green stem. Betony is often prescribed by herbalists to treat neuralgia, anxiety, migraine, gallstones, high blood pressure, and heartburn and to inhibit sweating. Also, it can be applied topically in an ointment to treat cuts and sores.

TIP: Betony is a bitter and aromatic herb, and it relieves gastritis, heartburn, and gas; improves appetite, and supports digestive health. To relieve acid reflux, use 2-4 drops of liquid extract or prepare a root decoction and have it once a day.

Availability: In most good herbal remedy stores. (e.g. iHerb.com, Amazon.com)

Antiviral Properties: Tannins, flavonoid glycosides, and stachydrine. Betony is *primarily used to fight the influenza virus.*

Collection & Preparation: Available as capsules, an extract, a tincture, or a tea. Can be made into a tea by mixing 1-2 tsp. of the dried root with boiling water.

Dosage: 2-6 mL of tincture 3 times a day mixed with water or 2-4 g of infusion, made by adding dried herb to boiling water for up to15 minutes, no more than 3 times per day.

Possible Side Effects: Stomach upset, diarrhea.

Contraindications: Do not take if you suffer from low blood pressure or if you're pregnant, breastfeeding, or trying to conceive.

Alternatives: Other herbs from the mint family, such as sage.

Other Uses: Asthma, Bronchitis, Headache, Digestive Problems, Intestinal Gas, Alzheimer's, Bladder and Kidney Stones.

32. Cardamom

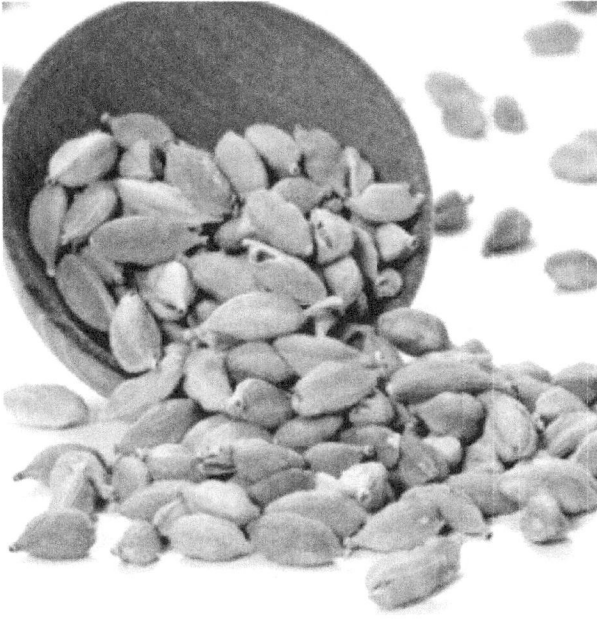

Cardamom belongs to the family Zingiberaceae and falls into two genera: Elettaria (Green) and Amomum (Black). This seed pod has long been popular due to its healing and culinary properties. Native to the evergreen rain forest in southern India, and the spice grows in certain tropical countries. Typically, the plant can reach 4 m in length and grows in thick clumps. It starts bearing the seed pods after approximately two years of plantation. Each pod can reach approximately 1-2 cm in length.

Both cardamom varieties produce three-sided pods covered by a papery thin, yet tough outer layer. Inside, tiny, aromatic seeds, ranging in color from deep brown to black, appear in vertical rows with a thin membrane covering each grain. Amomum pods appear large and dark brown, while Elettaria pods appear smaller and light green.

Black cardamom, *Amomum subulatum*, is also called Nepal cardamom ("bari" or "kali elaichi") and is a relatively bigger pod compared to Elettaria cardamom. The pod displays a rough, dark brown outer layer and can reach approximately 1-2 cm in diameter and 2-4 cm in length. These pods produce an intense, camphor-like flavor generally used in spicy stews in China and the sub-Himalayan plains of Pakistan, India, and Nepal.

TIP: Did you know that Cardamom is very effective in treating stress and depression? Crush Cardamom and put it in 1 cup of water. Boil on low flame, stain, and add a little honey. Drink it lukewarm once a day.

Availability: In most good health food and herbal remedy stores. (e.g. mountainroseherbs.com, iHerb.com, Amazon.com)

Antiviral Properties: Terpenes, which prevent viral cells from reproducing. Cardamom is *primarily used to help with digestive disorders.*

Collection & Preparation: Available as an oil, a tincture, a powder, or as food.

Dosage: The standard dosage is 1.5 g of the ground seeds per day or 1-2 g of tincture.

Possible Side Effects: Chest pains, throat tightness, shortness of breath, dermatitis, increased risk of bleeding, low blood pressure.

Contraindications: Do not take if you're suffering from gallstones, internal ulcers or if you are pregnant or breastfeeding.

Alternatives: Nutmeg.

Other Uses: Colic, Indigestion, IBS, Constipation, Depression, Liver and Kidney Problems, Bronchitis, Heartburn, Bad Breath, High Blood Pressure, Amebiasis, Cancer, Low Libido.

33. Chamomile

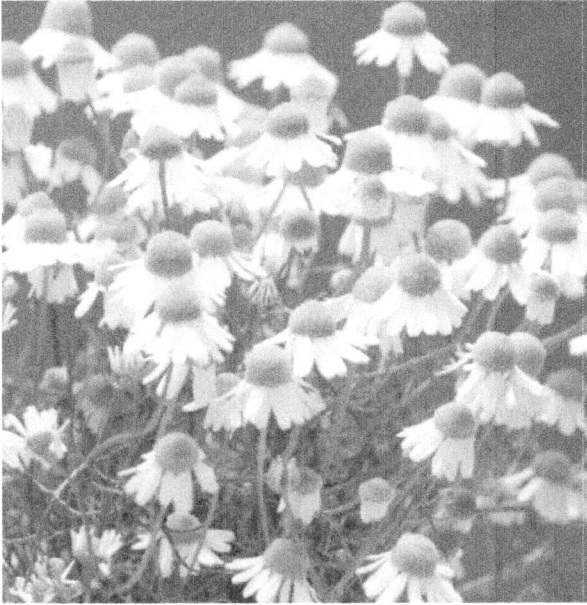

Chamomile is a popular medicinal herb, since ancient times, and the term actually describes a variety of daisy-like plants. They are members of the family Asteraceae, and there are various species. Two of the most common species are German chamomile, *Matricaria recutita*, and Roman chamomile, *Chamaemelum nobile*. They each provide unique health benefits, but both have been prized since ancient times in Rome, Greece, and Egypt for their anti-inflammatory and calming properties. Chamomile became even more popular through the Middle Ages as people started using it to treat numerous medical issues such as skin diseases, asthma, cancer, colic, nervous complaints, fevers, nausea, inflammation, and various children's ailments. In terms of being a popular remedy, it could be considered the European counterpart to Asian or Korean ginseng.

TIP: Chamomile is the best aid for irritated children. When the child wants a lap all the time and cries when put down for bed, or when one of his cheeks is red and hot, and the other is pale and cold, then prepare a little Chamomile tea and the child will calm down.

Availability: In most good health food and herbal remedy stores. (e.g. naturesremedy.co.uk, iHerb.com, Amazon.com)

Antiviral Properties: Terpenoids, flavonoids, coumarins, all of which reduce stress in the body. Chamomile is primarily *used for chickenpox and other similar skin viral conditions.*

Collection & Preparation: Available as a tablet, a capsule, a powder, a tincture, an oil, a cream, or a tea. The tea can be made by stewing Chamomile flowers in boiling water for 5-10 minutes.

Dosage: The standard capsule dosage is between 400 and 1,600 mg per day. It is recommended to drink between 1 and 4 cups of Chamomile tea per day.

Possible Side Effects: Drowsiness, dermatitis, diarrhea.

Contraindications: Do not take if you're using sedatives, blood thinners, pain killers or allergic to ragweed. Avoid if pregnant or nursing.

Alternatives: N/A.

Other Uses: Insomnia, Depression, Menstrual Cramps, Heartburn, Digestive Disorders, Dandruff, Vomiting, Colic, Skin Conditions, Gingivitis.

34. Cinnamon

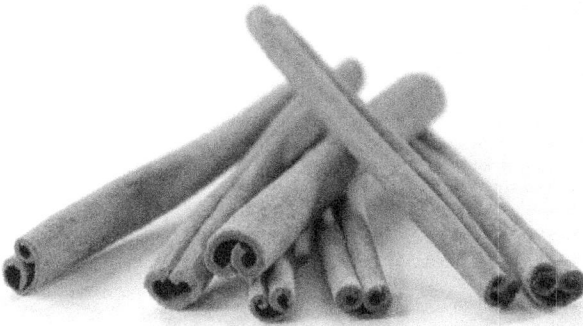

Cinnamon is a commonly used "warming" herb in Chinese medicine that supports digestion and circulation. It is a go-to ingredient for tea that is used to treat nausea during pregnancy and reduce hemorrhage after the baby's birth. This herb also promotes peripheral circulation, boosts vitality, fights congestion, warms the body systems, improves digestion, eases abdominal spasms, and stimulates the body's vital organs. Cinnamon comes from a small, evergreen tree in the family Lauraceae, where the spice is gathered from the dried inner bark of the tree's branches by peeling it off and letting the pieces dry and curl up. These dried pieces are the sticks used in cooking and herb teas.

TIP: Did you know that Cinnamon is a great herbal remedy to treat diabetes? Make a Cinnamon infusion by soaking pieces overnight in a bowl of water. Drink the infusion half an hour before your first meal of the day.

Availability: In most good health food and herbal remedy stores. (e.g. healthspan.co.uk, iHerb.com, Amazon.com)

Antiviral Properties: Volatile oils, which prevent viral cells from reproducing. Cinnamon is *primarily used to fight influenza*.

Collection & Preparation: Can be taken as a juice, powder or prepared with food. Also can be bought as tablets and capsules.

Dosage: 1-6 g per day for no longer than 6 weeks.

Possible Side Effects: Increased heart rate and palpitations.

Contraindications: Do not take if using blood thinners such as *Warfarin*. Also avoid it if you experience prostate problems.

Alternatives: N/A.

Other Uses: Improving Glucose and Lipid Levels, Gout, High Blood Pressure, HIV, Multiple Sclerosis.

35. Clove

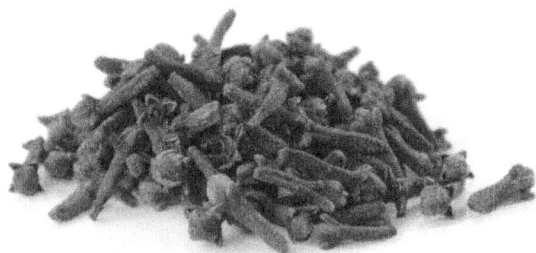

Cloves, *Syzygium aromaticum*, are among the highly revered spices, with culinary and healing properties that are recognized across the globe. This spice is technically the "flower buds" blooming on an evergreen tree belonging to the family Myrtaceae and native to rain forests in Indonesia. The buds start out pale in color, then eventually turn green. By the time they are harvested, the cloves will develop into their distinct bright red. Mature buds achieve nearly 2 cm in length before they are picked.

TIP: Clove is a great herbal treatment for toothache and gingivitis. It can also help to get rid of bad breath and dry mouth or diminish cavities. For toothache, chew 2 Cloves and apply around the sore teeth. If you prefer to use essential oil, add 1 drop to a cotton ball then place around the sore teeth.

Availability: In most good health food and herbal remedy stores. (e.g. newwayherbs.com, iHerb.com, Amazon.com)

Antiviral Properties: Carvacrol, thymol, eugenol, and cinnamaldehyde. Cloves are *primarily used to fight the common cold and respiratory disorders.*

Collection & Preparation: Buy whole Cloves rather than powder, store them in a cool, dark place, and cook them with your food. Also available as an oil or essential oil.

Dosage: *For toothache* – put 2-3 drops of Clove oil in 1 cup of warm water. Gargle 3-4 times a day. *For bloating* – take 4-5 drops of Clove oil in a glass of water and drink it twice a day.

Possible Side Effects: Dermatitis, vomiting, dizziness, diarrhea, and bloating.

Contraindications: Do not use if allergic to eugenol, suffer from Crohn's disease, or have liver problems. Avoid use of Cloves and Clove oil during pregnancy. Can also cause irritation if used in its pure form.

Alternatives: Basil, marjoram, cinnamon.

Other Uses: Digestion Issues, Lack of Appetite, Travel Sickness, Respiration Diseases, Acid Reflux, Candidiasis.

36. Oregon Grape Root (Creeping Mahonia)

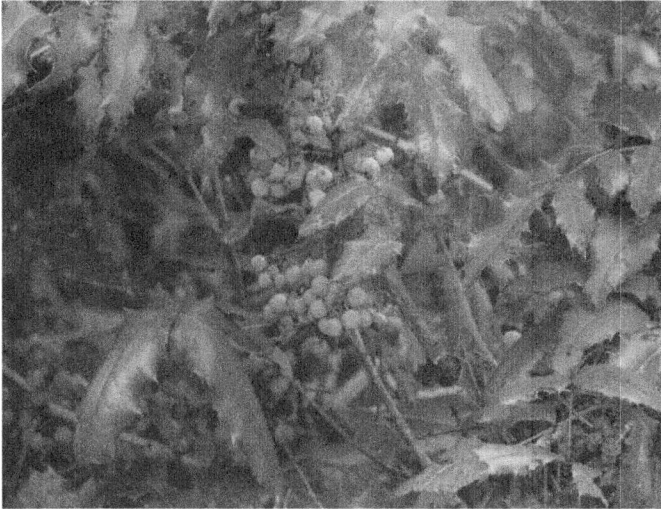

Oregon Grape is applied to treat those diagnosed with cold sores, acne, psoriasis and eczema, and acute and chronic urinary tract infections. The roots and stems are the medicinal parts of this plant, and the best time to harvest is during the early spring, fall, and winter. Wait for the berries to fall off, but don't wait so long that new leaves sprout. Holding out for this particular period makes sure the medicinal properties of the plant are concentrated below the soil. Then, scrape the medicinal bark off the roots and stems to be used fresh in tinctures or later after being dried to make infusions.

Availability: Available in most good herbal remedy shops. (e.g. iHerb.com, Amazon.com)

Antiviral Properties: Isoquinoline alkaloids berberine and hydrazine. Oregon Grape Root is *primarily used for cytomegalovirus, human papillomavirus, and the herpes simplex virus.*

Collection & Preparation: Available as a cream, an extract, a tincture, or capsules. Can also be made into a tea by simmering 1-2 tsp. of coarsely cut root for 10-15 minutes.

Dosage: Take for no longer than 1 week, leaving at least a 7-day break. *For infection* – take as an infusion: 5-15 g of chopped roots boiled in 2 cups of water for 15 minutes. Infused and strained, can be taken in up to 3 cups a day.

Possible Side Effects: Can cause jaundice and kernicterus in children. May cause diarrhea, kidney irritation, liver toxicity, nausea.

Contraindications: Do not take while pregnant or breastfeeding or suffering from diarrhea or liver disease. Not recommended for children.

Alternatives: Barberry, coptis, goldenseal.

Other Uses: Stomach Ulcers, Psoriasis, Blood Impurity, Dysentery, Eczema, Syphilis, Rheumatism, Reflux.

37. Ginger

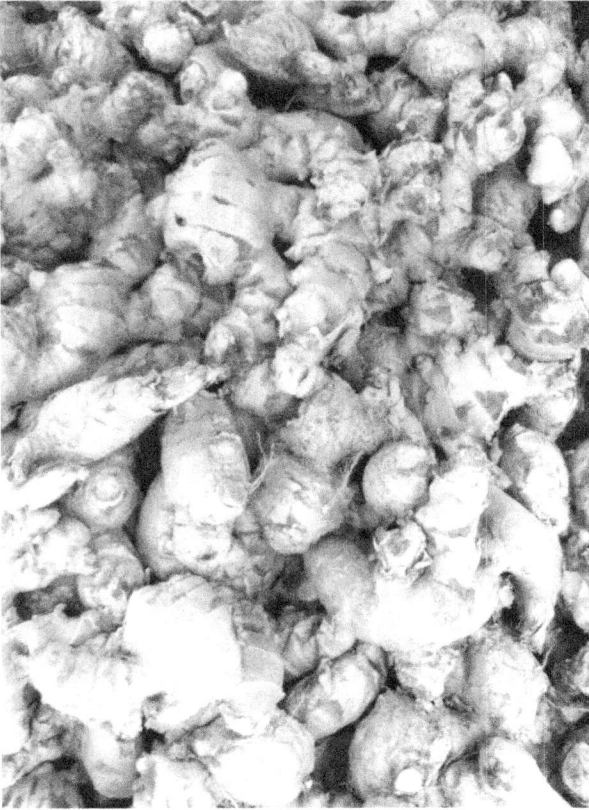

Ginger is typically applied by herbalists to treat digestive problems, but it is also used to alleviate arthritis, motion sickness, and symptoms of the common cold. This spice has made a regular appearance in Asian cuisine for over five thousand years, but, in China, history of its use strictly as a remedy has lasted over two thousand years. Later on, Europeans believed its power came from the Garden of Eden, and early American settlers used it as an ingredient in beer.

TIP: Did you know that Ginger is effective in cases of premenstrual syndrome? Use Ginger root to make a tea and take it twice a day, or chew a piece of fresh Ginger. It will help to relieve the symptoms associated with PMS by soothing cramps, relieving nausea, and reducing mood swings and fatigue.

Availability: In most good health food and herbal remedy stores. (e.g. naturesbest.co.uk, iHerb.com, Amazon.com)

Antiviral Properties: Rhizome and flavonoids, which protect healthy cells, preventing virus reproduction. Ginger is *primarily used to fight off influenza.*

Collection & Preparation: Can be bought as food, drinks, sweets, capsules, tinctures, and tablets. Ginger can be made into a tea by mixing 1 tbsp. of fresh grated Ginger with boiling water.

Dosage: Capsules or tablets – 250 mg 4 times a day. Avoid excessive consumption.

Possible Side Effects: Heartburn, stomach discomfort, extra menstrual bleeding, irritation. May cause high blood pressure if taken in high dosage.

Contraindications: Do not take if using *Warfarin*, diabetes medication, heart medication, or aspirin. Avoid Ginger oil during pregnancy.

Alternatives: Honey.

Other Uses: Hay Fever, Allergies, Nausea, Vomiting, Cancer, Diabetics, Ulcers, Gastric Distress, Inflammation, Radiation, High Blood Pressure, Arthritis, Angina.

Ginger root (raw)

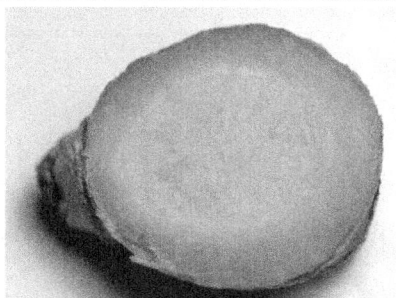

Ginger section

Nutritional value per 100 g (3.5 oz)

Energy	333 kJ (80 kcal)	
Carbohydrates	17.77 g	
Sugars	1.7 g	
Dietary fiber	2 g	
Fat	0.75 g	
Protein	1.82 g	
Vitamins	**Quantity**	**%DV**[†]
Thiamine (B$_1$)	0.025 mg	2%
Riboflavin (B$_2$)	0.034 mg	3%
Niacin (B$_3$)	0.75 mg	5%
Pantothenic acid (B$_5$)	0.203 mg	4%
Vitamin B$_6$	0.16 mg	12%
Folate (B$_9$)	11 µg	3%
Vitamin C	5 mg	6%
Vitamin E	0.26 mg	2%
Minerals	**Quantity**	**%DV**[†]
Calcium	16 mg	2%
Iron	0.6 mg	5%
Magnesium	43 mg	12%
Manganese	0.229 mg	11%
Phosphorus	34 mg	5%
Potassium	415 mg	9%
Sodium	13 mg	1%
Zinc	0.34 mg	4%
Other constituents	**Quantity**	
Water	79 g	

38. Oregano

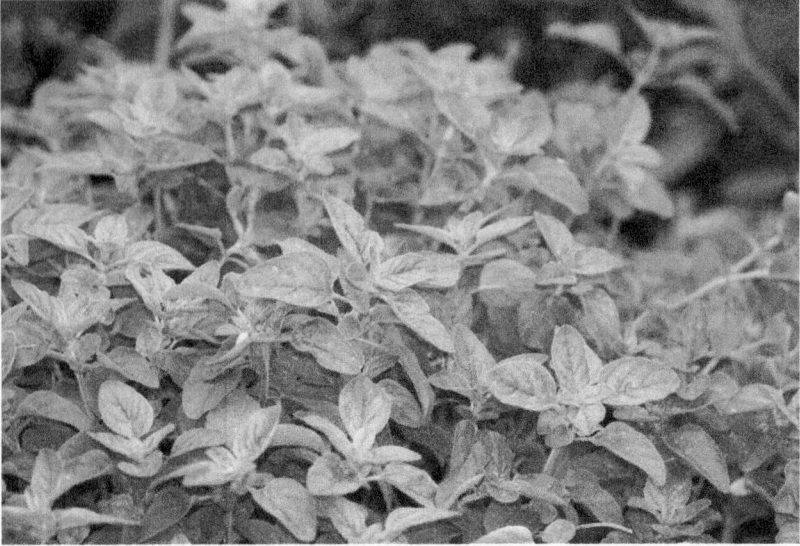

Oregano is a naturally therapeutic herb with potent phytochemicals providing health benefits whether it is used in your cooking or directly as a medicinal supplement. Popular in Mediterranean dishes, and known most for the flavor it brings to pizza sauce, oregano adds Vitamins A, B6, C, E, and K to your diet, along with potassium, calcium, fiber, magnesium, iron, and folate. It is also known as "*wild marjoram*" throughout Europe due to its relation to sweet marjoram, but oregano means "mountain joy" and the ancient Romans and Greeks revered the herb as a symbol of happiness. In fact, drawings from those times depict the tradition of brides and grooms wearing a laurel of oregano like a crown.

TIP: Oregano actively fights against infections and several skin-related problems, including acne. It can give you smooth and infection-free skin. Add 2 drops of Oregano oil in 1 tbsp. of coconut or olive oil and massage the affected areas.

Availability: Most good herbal remedy and health food shops. (e.g. puritan.com, iHerb.com, Amazon.com)

Antiviral Properties: Terpenes and thymol, which fight off viral infections. Oregano is *primarily used for respiratory tract infections.*

Collection & Preparation: It can be used in food or bought as an oil, a cream, or capsules.

Dosage: Use 1 part Oregano oil diluted with 2 parts olive oil for external use. For internal use, take 2-3 drops of Oregano oil in 1 cup of water.

Possible Side Effects: Can cause a reaction if you're allergic to plants in the Lamiaceae family. It may also cause skin irritation and stomach upset.

Contraindications: Do not take if you suffer from bleeding disorders or diabetes. Avoid use in pregnancy and while breastfeeding.

Alternatives: N/A.

Other Uses: Muscle Pain, Norovirus, Herpes Simplex Virus, Athlete's Foot, Dandruff, Wrinkles, Asthma, Cuts and Bruises, Earaches, Influenza, Acne, Varicose Veins.

39. Acacia (Catechu)

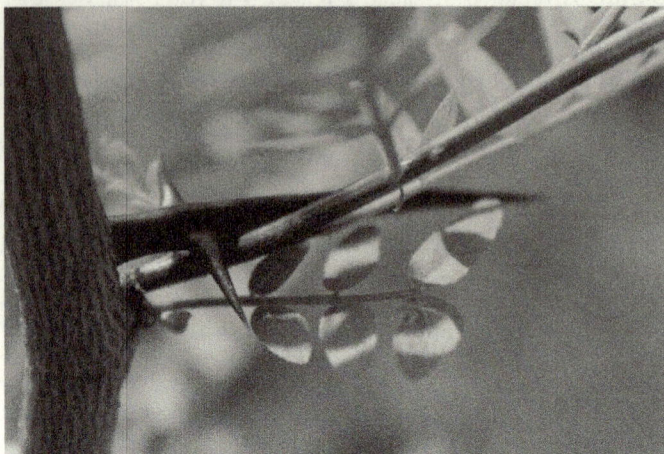

For thousands of years, Acacia trees have been known for their medicinal properties, decorative uses, and strong wood. Today, Acacia's popularity has grown due to renewed focus on its medicinal properties and recommendations from herbalist experts to use it as a natural remedy to alleviate a wide variety of disorders. It's said that Hebrews have long considered the wood of the acacia tree sacred and that a legend exists stating Christ's crown of thorns had come from an acacia tree.

TIP: Acacia can help you get rid of parasitic roundworms, e.g. ascaris. Drink 26 mL bark decoction of catechu 2 times a day.

Availability: In most good herbal remedy stores. (e.g. iHerb.com, Amazon.com)

Antiviral Properties: Taxifolin, which fights viral cells. Acacia is *primarily used to cure human papillomavirus.*

Collection & Preparation: Available as seeds, a powder, in honey, and a gum that needs to be combined with water to work successfully.

Dosage: 5 g of powder twice a day for 4-6 weeks.

Possible Side Effects: Gas, bloating, nausea and loose stools, hypotension, asthma, rhinitis.

Contraindications: Do not take if pregnant or breastfeeding.

Alternatives: N/A.

Other Uses: Weight Loss Aid, Throat and Stomach Inflammation, Skin Diseases, Eyes Bloodshot, Anemia.

40. Goldenseal

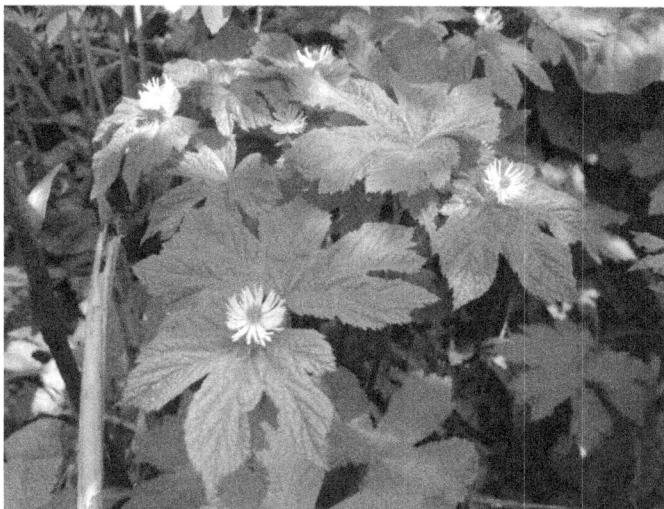

Goldenseal is known for its ability to stimulate the body's immune system, and so, it has been used medicinally throughout history. This herb is believed to have powerful antiviral properties, making it popular for use against the flu and common cold. It can be consumed as a tea or used as a topical wash and gargle to treat herpes lesions and cold sores. Due to extreme harvesting in the wild, this bushy plant is considered an endangered species. Before this, it generously grew in the wild within rich soils; it displays bright yellow flowers that generate a beautiful red oil upon infusion.

TIP: Goldenseal has strong antibacterial and antiseptic properties that help to reduce inflammation in the prostate. Goldenseal soothes the urinary tract and treats prostatitis. Add 2-3 tsp. of dried Goldenseal flower in 1 cup of hot water and boil it for 5 minutes on a medium flame. Strain well and drink twice a day.

Availability: In most good herbal remedy stores. (e.g. iHerb.com, Amazon.com)

Antiviral Properties: Berberine and isoquinoline alkaloids, which work to inhibit viral cells. Goldenseal *primarily fights influenza.*

Collection & Preparation: Available as a tablet, a capsule, an extract, or a tincture.

Dosage: 0.5-1 g tablets or capsules, 0.3-1 ml of liquid/fluid extract, or 10-20 drops of tincture – all taken 2-3 times a day. Do not take on an empty stomach.

Possible Side Effects: Numbness, sickness, diarrhea, allergic reactions on skin, or throat problems.

Contraindications: Do not use if pregnant, breastfeeding or on newborn babies. Avoid using if the following health issues exist: blood pressure problems, heart problems, diabetes, glaucoma. Avoid use if allergic to ragweed. Consult a doctor before taking it.

Alternatives: Oregon Grape Root.

Other Uses: Food Poisoning, Eczema, Cough, Sinusitis, Constipation, Cancer, Hay Fever, Hemorrhoids, Chronic Fatigue, Liver Problems, Arrhythmia, Prostatitis.

41. Juniper

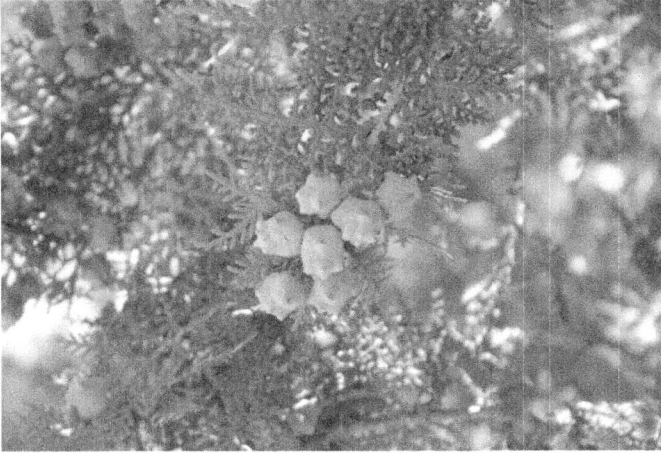

Juniper, *Juniperus communis*, has natural antiseptic, antibacterial, diuretic, and antiviral properties. The medicinal part of the evergreen trees, blue-black scales from the tree's cones, known as the "berries," are popular to treat a variety of health conditions. It has provided support during childbirth and been a remedy for infectious diseases.

Juniper grows wild in regions of North America, Asia, and Europe. *Juniperus communis* is the most common variety of juniper in North America, among the many out there. This particular variety can reach 10 ft tall and displays seed cones and leaves that resemble needles. Scales from the cones of the male juniper take 18 months to ripen, while the scales of a female juniper take 2-3 years to ripen.

TIP: Juniper berries extract has anti-inflammatory properties. It gives relief from the pain associated with arthritis, rheumatism, and gout. The joint pain causes fluid retention and pressure in the joints. Juniper extract eases this pain.

Availability: In most good herbal remedy stores. (e.g. naturessunshine.com, iHerb.com, Amazon.com)

Antiviral Properties: Amentoflavone, which prevents viral cells from reproducing. Juniper is *primarily used for viral gastroenteritis*.

Collection & Preparation: Available as an oil, a tincture, a tablet, a capsule, or berries that can be used in food.

Dosage: 20-100 mg of the essential oil, 2-10 g of the berries daily.

Possible Side Effects: Skin and respiratory allergic reactions can occur. It may also cause stomach upset.

Contraindications: Do not use if pregnant or breastfeeding. Avoid use if you suffer from diabetes, kidney diseases, stomach and intestinal disorders, or blood pressure issues.

Alternatives: N/A.

Other Uses: Heartburn, Indigestion, Urinary Tract Infections, Asthma, Bronchitis, Joint Pain, Kidney and Bladder Stones, Skin Problems.

42. Sage

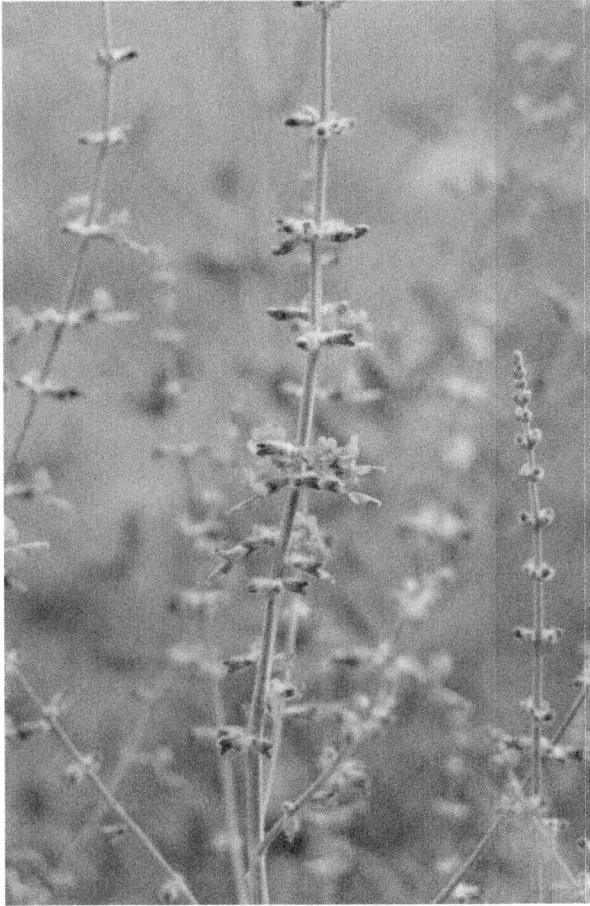

Sage is an herb with medicinal properties that help relieve the symptoms of digestive problems and mental disorders, such as depression and Alzheimer's. Native to the Mediterranean and belonging to the family Lamiaceae (mint), along with basil, oregano, rosemary, lavender, and thyme, this herb displays gray leaves that can reach 2.5 in and pink, white, purple, or blue flowers. Sage is popular for use in cosmetics and soaps because of its pleasant, distinct aroma.

TIP: Sage is beneficial in reducing the heavy perspiration of night sweats and hot flashes. It is also an old remedy for drying up breast milk. However, it works best for stomach problems – it keeps the stomach, intestines, kidneys, liver, and sexual organs healthy.

Availability: In most good herbal remedy stores. (e.g. <u>healthspan.co.uk</u>, iHerb.com, Amazon.com)

Antiviral Properties: Tannins and flavonoids, which inhibit viral cells. Sage is *primarily used for influenza, but is extremely beneficial in fighting the herpes simplex virus.*

Collection & Preparation: Available as a capsule, a tablet, an extract, an essential oil, a cream, or an herb for food. Can be made into a tea by placing 1 tsp. of powdered or fresh Sage in boiling water. Can be made into a tonic by pouring 1 qt. of boiling water over a handful of leaves and allow it to stew overnight.

Dosage: 1-2.5 g of dried Sage leaf or its equivalent 3 times a day.

Possible Side Effects: Restlessness, irritability, headaches, stomach upset and dizziness, epilepsy.

Contraindications: Do not use if you suffer from diabetes, epilepsy, high blood pressure, or seizure disorders; also if pregnant or breastfeeding.

Alternatives: Rosemary.

Other Uses: Sore Throat, Stomach Pain, Difficult Menses, Cold, Menopause Side Effects, Bloating, Memory Loss, Overproduction of Saliva, Alzheimer's.

43. Greater Celandine

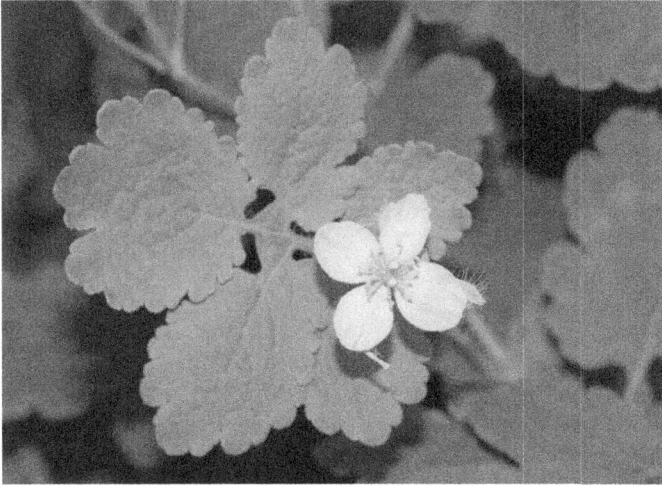

Greater celandine, *Chelidonium majus*, has long been used in several European countries. Dioscorides, Pliny the Elder, and the ancient Greeks in general described Celandine as a reliable detoxifying agent. For the Romans, Celandine was employed as a blood cleanser. French herbalist Maurice Mességué touted Celandine tea for treatment of liver problems. Traditional Chinese medicine and Western phytotherapy also praise its healing properties. Greater Celandine extracts have exhibited the capacity to protect the liver and a notable toxicity toward harmful organisms. Such a capacity has generated interest in employing Greater Celandine as a major aspect of protocols supporting and cleansing the gallbladder and liver.

TIP: This herb is very effective in treating warts. Keep in mind, though, the fresh juice can be toxic and could blister your skin, so dab no more than 3 warts at the same time with a cotton ball no more than 3 times a day.

Availability: In most good herbal remedy stores. (e.g. iHerb.com, Amazon.com)

Antiviral Properties: Alkaloids and flavonoids, which work to fight and kill viral cells. Greater Celandine is *primarily used for viral hepatitis*.

Collection & Preparation: Available as a cream or a tincture. The roots are used to create this medicine.

Dosage: The cream can be applied as needed. Take the tincture in 10-20 drops twice a day for 4 weeks.

Possible Side Effects: The cream can cause a skin rash. High dosage can cause breathing problems, sleepiness, and coughing.

Contraindications: Do not use if you suffer from autoimmune diseases, diarrhea, liver disease, hepatitis or if you have a bile duct blockage. Avoid giving to children, and avoid use if pregnant or breastfeeding.

Alternatives: N/A.

Other Uses: Jaundice, High Blood Pressure, Hepatitis, Cancer, Anxiety, Arthritis, Warts, IBS, Constipation, Menstrual Cramps, Pain.

44. Neem (Margosa)

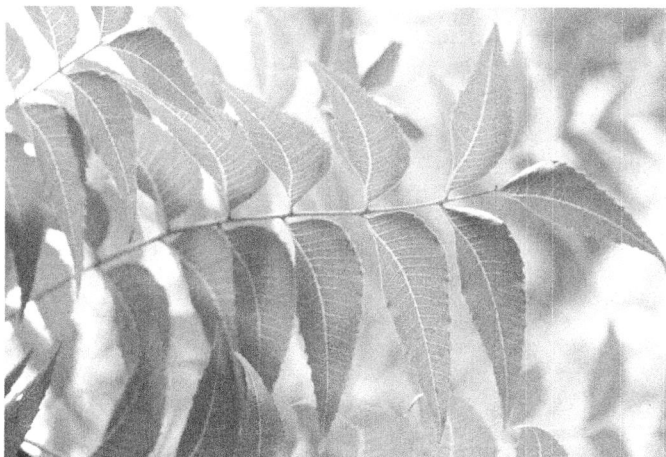

The last fifty years has seen the expansion of neem tree products beyond Asia and into other parts of the world, allowing American and European scientists to study its potential medical benefits. This ancient tree from Asia has been a source of medicinal extracts for centuries. Bearing a history that extends to the beginning of Hinduism, the neem tree continues to be a valuable herbal remedy for daily life and alleviating various irritants and ailments. India's history has documented farmers who purposefully grew neem trees for the medicinal benefits as early as the Vedic period, 1500-600 BC. Neem has also been used medicinally in India within traditional Ayurvedic herbal healing treatments. As people learn more about Neem and studies provide positive results about its use, this ancient herbal remedy can become a more widely accepted aspect of daily health regimens.

TIP: People with chickenpox are recommended to sleep on Neem leaves. You can also add some Neem leaves into your bathing water.

Availability: In most good herbal remedy stores. (e.g. theneemteam.co.uk, iHerb.com, Amazon.com)

Antiviral Properties: Polyphenolics such as flavonoids and their glycosides, dihydrochalcone, coumarin, and tannins, which interact with the surface of the viral cells to stop them from reproducing. Neem is *primarily used for the herpes, chickenpox, and hepatitis viruses.*

Collection & Preparation: Available as an oil, an extract, a tincture, capsules, and a tea by mixing the leaves with boiling water.

Dosage: Capsules = 1-2 twice a day and oil/tincture = 5 drops daily.

Possible Side Effects: If taken for a long period of time, it can harm your kidneys and liver. Can cause stomach irritation.

Contraindications: Do not use if you are trying to conceive; or suffer from autoimmune disorders, diabetes; or have had an organ transplant. Avoid if pregnant or breastfeeding.

Alternatives: N/A.

Other Uses: Leprosy, Dandruff, Eye Disorders, Gum Disease, Hemorrhoids, Blood Vessels.

45. Sanguinaria (Bloodroot)

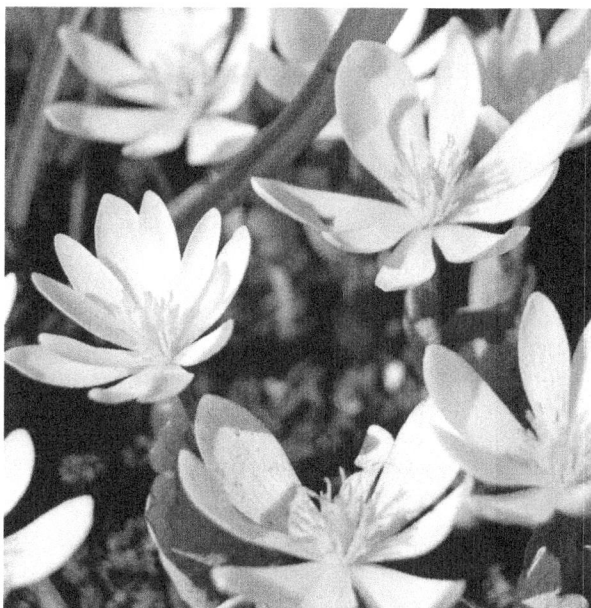

Sanguinaria is an extract taken from the root of the *Sanguinaria canadensis* and *Poppy fumaria* species. It is a plant alkaloid shown to possess antioxidant, antimicrobial, and anti-inflammatory properties. Due to those properties, it is popular as a toothpaste additive and an antiseptic mouth rinse to inhibit dental plaque and gingival inflammation. Sanguinaria is defined as a cationic molecule, which means that it converts to an alkanolamine form at a pH greater than 7 from an iminium ion form at a pH less than 6. Sanguinaria has been found to impede platelet aggregation caused by a sub-threshold concentration of thrombin, arachidonic acid, and collagen.

TIP: Did you know that Bloodroot is the key ingredient in herbal tooth-pastes and mouth rinse? It prevents tooth decay and other gum diseases, protects from gingivitis, and gives relief from severe tooth ache.

Availability: In most good herbal remedy stores. (e.g. iHerb.com, Amazon.com)

Antiviral Properties: Alkaloids sanguinarine and berberine, which kill off viral cells. Sanguinaria is *primarily used to fight HIV or warts.*

Collection & Preparation: Available as a tincture, a powder, toothpaste, and a fluid.

Dosage: Tincture = 10-15 drops, powder = 1 grain, and fluid = 10-30 drops daily.

Possible Side Effects: Nausea, vomiting, drowsiness, vertigo, burning in the stomach, low blood pressure.

Contraindications: Do not use if you suffer from intestinal problems or glaucoma. Avoid if pregnant or breastfeeding.

Alternatives: N/A.

Other Uses: Croup, Bronchitis, Skin Problems, Warts, Nasal Polyps, Achy Joints, Gum Disease, Poor Circulation, High Blood Pressure, Headache, Cancer.

Of course, there are many amazing herbs with great antiviral uses and other health benefits. This list is just the start of the things that can help you! Further research can assist you if it is an area of your interest. There are many online resources with information, some of which are listed later in this guide.

Tip: iHerb.com has most of the herbal antivirals you may need for very affordable prices. Make sure to take advantage of $5 off for the first order with the following voucher code: **WCR736**.

CHAPTER 6
LITTLE KNOWN HERBAL REMEDY RECIPES

There are many antiviral recipes that you can create in your own home. Here are some brilliant ones that are easy to create and work to **fight the symptoms of influenza**:

1. Ginger, Garlic, and Onion Soup – *for the common cold.*

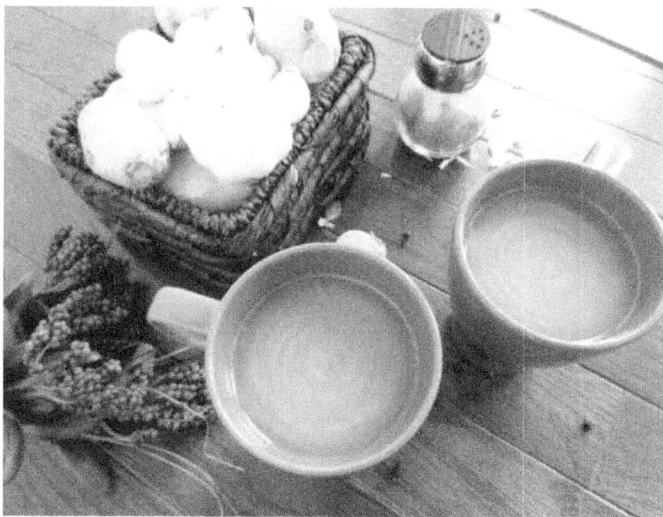

- ⅓ cup each of chopped Ginger, Garlic, and Onion
- 2 cups of pure Water

Mix ingredients together and boil on a high heat for 20 minutes, before simmering for another 10. Strain to complete the soup. Drink this as often as you like.

2. Cinnamon and Elderberry Soup – *for bronchitis.*

- 1 cup of Elderberries
- 1 cup of organic Honey
- 1 Cinnamon stick
- 5 Cloves
- 1 Star Anise (*obtained from the star-shaped Illicium Verum fruit found in China*)
- 1 tsp. of Orange, Lemon, or Lime zest
- ⅓ cup of grated organic Ginger
- 2 cups of Water

Simmer all ingredients in a small pan for 40 minutes until the liquid is well reduced. Once you have strained the liquid, and while it's all warm, stir in the honey. Take 1 tsp. of this every morning and night until you feel better.

3. 'The Master Tonic' – *for influenza.*

- 1 cup of fresh chopped Garlic
- 1 cup of fresh chopped Onion
- 1 cup of fresh grated Ginger Root
- 1 cup of fresh grated Horseradish Root
- 1 cup of chopped fresh Cayenne Peppers
- Raw, unfiltered Apple Cider Vinegar

Mix the chopped vegetables and grated herbs together and then top it with the apple cider vinegar. Shake this tonic at least once a day for 2 weeks before consuming and then drink 2 or more times daily (1 or 2 oz.) until you're well. For infections – dose must be taken 5-6 times a day. *It is safe during pregnancy and for children (in small doses).*

4. Basic Cold & Flu Tea – *for cold and flu symptoms.*

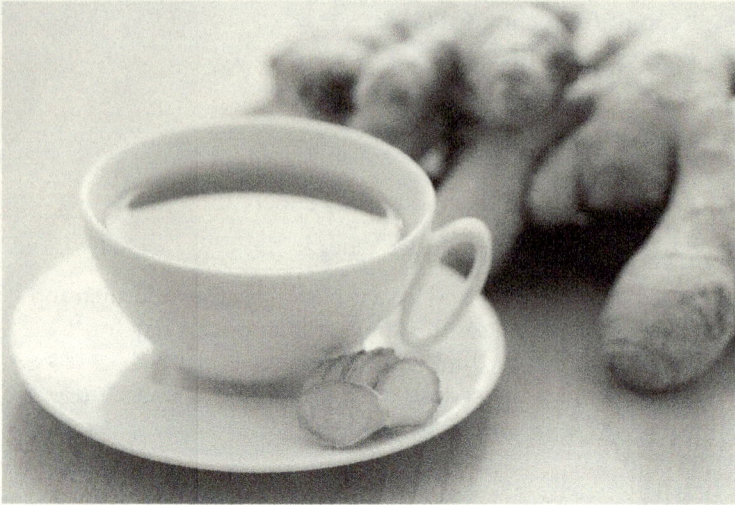

- 3-4 Ginger slices, unpeeled
- 1 Garlic clove, chopped
- Tea (green, oolong, black, or your preference)
- Cayenne Powder
- Milk
- Honey

In a sauce pan with water, bring garlic and ginger to a boil. Allow to simmer about 20 minutes. Using garlic-ginger water, steep tea. Flavor with cayenne powder just hot enough to induce sweating. Add milk and honey to taste. You can drink up to 4 cups per day, especially before bed, where bundling up can help induce sweating.

5. Garlic Lemonade – *for influenza.*

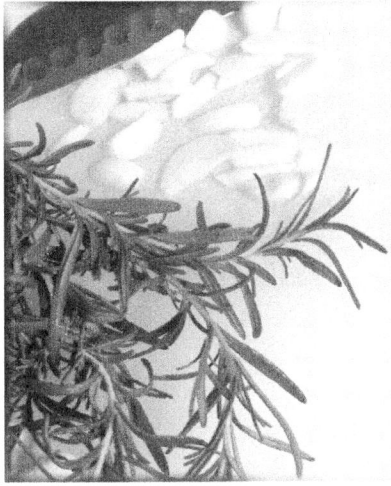

- 2-4 cloves chopped Garlic
- 3-4 slices of chopped Ginger
- 2-3 Lemons
- Honey
- Water

Find a 1 qt. mason jar, and then combine water, ginger, and garlic inside. Cover the water, ginger, and garlic, allowing them to steep for 20 minutes, at least. Add honey (about ¼ cup) and the juice from the lemons to taste. Keep the herbs in or filter them out of the mixture at your preference. Drink warm or at room temperature (but not cold) and whenever it's needed.

6. Lemon Balm Home Remedy – *for cold sores and herpes virus.*

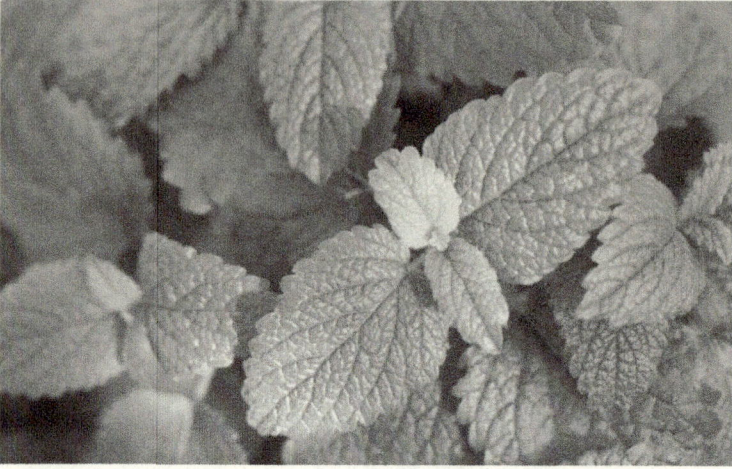

- 2 tsp. Lemon Balm, dried (or 2 Lemon Balm teabags)
- 1 cup of Water, boiling

Pour boiling water over lemon balm and steep for up to15 minutes, then strain. Dab a cotton ball in the mixture and apply it to the cold sore 4 times a day or more. You could also drink lemon balm tea to help fight the virus.

7. Onion and Honey Cough Medicine – *for coughs.*

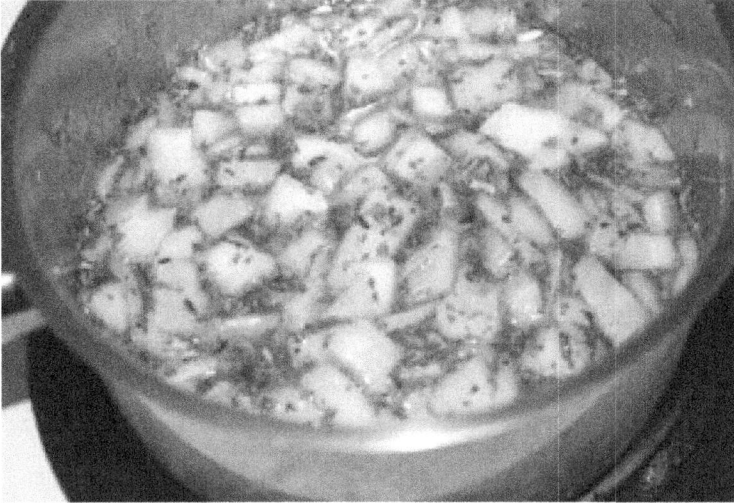

- 1 cup Onion, chopped
- ½ cup Honey
- 1-2 tbsp. Cloves, Marshmallow Root, and Ginger (flavor to your preference)

Add chopped onions plus the herbs of your choice into a small glass or stainless-steel pot. Coat the herbs and onions with honey.

Slowly simmer mixture in pot on low heat. Keep the temperature low; allow the honey to soften and the herbs to steep. Use a lid during this process to help retain the medicinal properties of the syrup's herbs. Do remove the lid every few minutes to give it a quick stir and make sure it doesn't burn.

Let the mixture simmer about 20 minutes and remove from heat. Strain out the herbs and onions. Store the remaining liquid (which might contain remnants of the herbs) in a small glass jar with a lid and refrigerate. Take as needed (*1 tsp. for children and 1 tbsp. for anyone above 10 years*).

8. Cinnamon Licorice Tea – *for coronavirus (boosting energy during healing).*

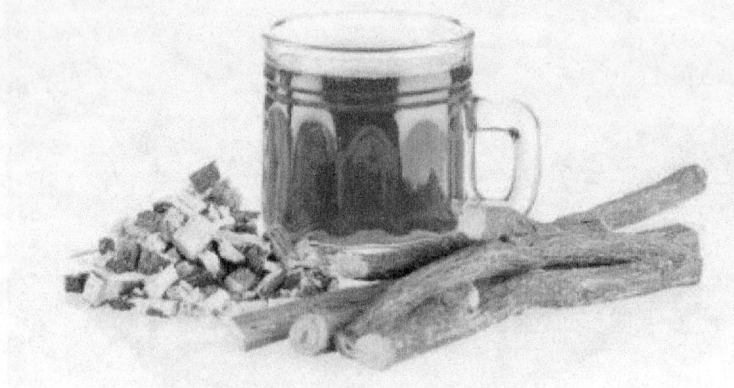

- 2 quarts Water (purified)
- 2 tbsp. Astragalus Root
- 1 tsp. Licorice Root
- 1 stick of Cinnamon

Break the cinnamon into pieces and combine it with the licorice, astragalus, and water in a pot. Bring to a boil, cover, and allow it to steep for about 3 minutes on a warm surface. You can use a wood stove, but the lowest heat on an ordinary stove works well also.

When ready, let it sit for a couple of hours. Reheat it and drink one glass, once or twice per day.

9. Thyme Tea – *for coronavirus (fever and cough symptoms).*

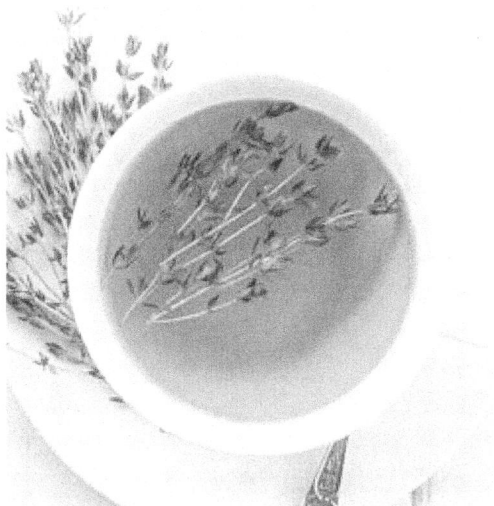

- 3 sprigs Thyme (fresh; substitute: 2 sprigs Thyme, dried)
- 1 ½cup Water

Put the thyme sprigs in a teacup and add boiling water. Cover and allow to steep for about 5 minutes. Remove the sprigs before you drink.

10. Turmeric and Ginger Hot Cider Tea – *for coronavirus (dry coughs and fever).*

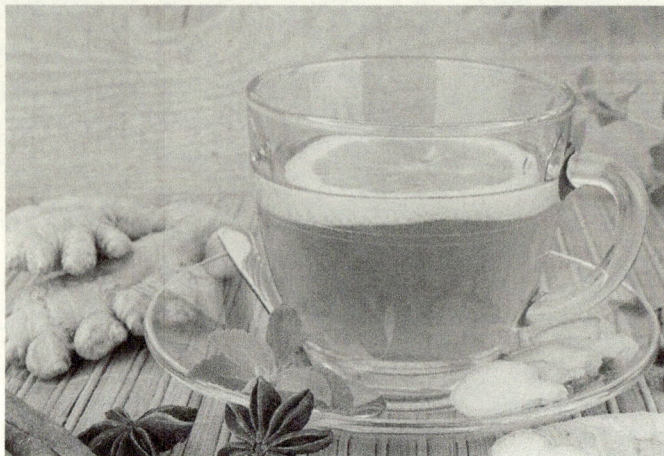

- 1 cup Apple Cider (sweet, fresh)
- 1 tsp. Turmeric (grated, fresh)
- 1 tsp. Ginger (grated, fresh)
- 1 Lemon Peel (½ inch x ½ inch strip, include white part)

Add the ginger, cider, lemon peel, and turmeric in a small saucepan set over medium heat, combine and heat. When a ring of bubbles starts appearing around the edge of your pan, cover and set aside to steep for about 5 minutes.

Pour into a mug through a fine tea strainer and serve immediately.

11. **Neem Recipe** – *for chickenpox.*

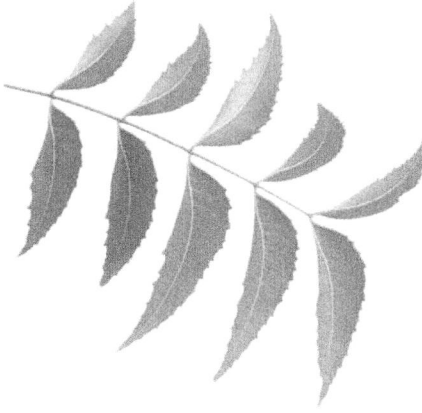

- Neem leaves
- Water

Crush the neem leaves in the water and create a paste. Apply this paste topically to the affected area. Prepare a neem bath after the disease is cured, when the scabs have fallen away from the skin. Add the leaves to bathwater and soak.

CHAPTER 7

HERBAL REMEDIES FOR COMMON AILMENTS

Ailment	Herb
Acne	Aloe vera, oregano, echinacea
Allergy	Chamomile, turmeric, ginger
Anxiety and stress	Hops, kava, passionflower, valerian, chamomile, lavender
Asthma	Coffee, ephedra, echinacea, cat's claw
Bad breath/body odor	Alfalfa, billberry, clove
Bloating	Basil, cilantro, peppermint, sage
Bronchitis	Echinacea, pelargonium, red root, cat's claw
Colds	Echinacea, andrographis, ginseng, licorice root (sore throat), astragalus root, garlic, turmeric
Cough	Eucalyptus, basil, goldenseal, red root
Dizziness	Ginger, ginkgo
Digestive problems	Alfalfa, basil, bee balm, billberry, oregano
Earache	Echinacea, oregano, basil

Fatigue	Cocoa (dark chocolate), coffee, eleutheroccocus, ginseng, rhodiola, cat's claw, goldenseal
Flu	Echinacea, elderberry syrup (also see "Colds")
Hay fever	Stinging nettle, butterbur, ginger, perilla
Herpes	Topical lemon balm, topical comfrey, echinacea, garlic, ginseng, basil, oregano, fennel
Hot flashes	Red clover, soy, black cohosh, sage
Infection	Topical tea tree oil, astragalus, echinacea, eleutherococcus, garlic, ginseng, rhodiola
Insomnia	Catnip, cilantro, chamomile
Joint pain	Ashwagandha, dandelion, juniper, pau d'arco
Malaria	Boneset, basil, cordyceps, pau d'arco
Migraine	Feverfew, butterbur, bearberry, peppermint, betony
Muscle pain	Capsicum, wintergreen, rosemary, oregano
Nausea	Ginger, peppermint, Oregon grape
Sore throat	Licorice, marshmallow, mullein, bee balm, sage
Stuffy nose	Echinacea
Tonsillitis	Goldenseal, astragalus, echinacea, red root
Toothache	Willow, clove oil, coriander

SOURCES

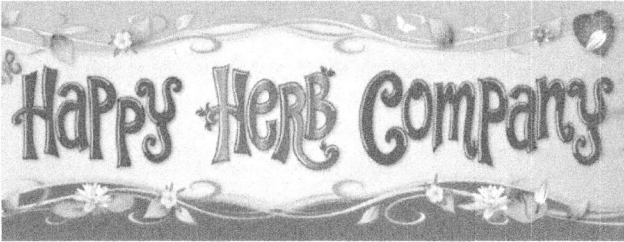

happyherbcompany.com

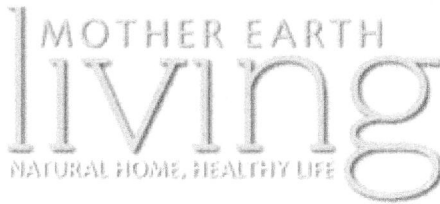

motherearthliving.com

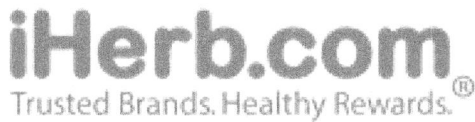

iherb.com

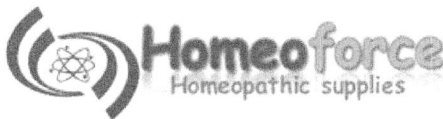

homeoforce.co.uk

nelsonsnaturalworld.com

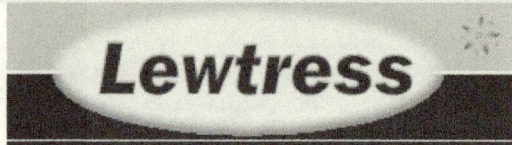

lewtress-health.com

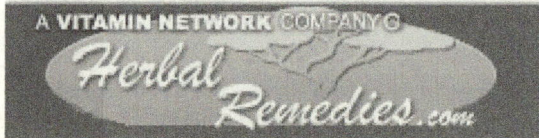

herbalremedies.com

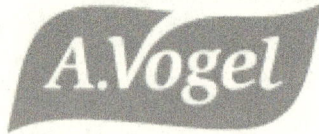

avogel.com

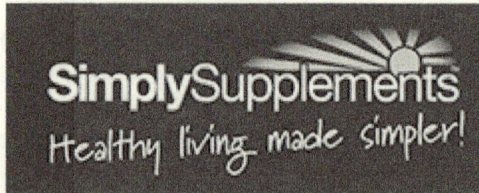

simplysupplements.net

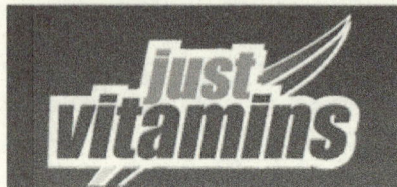

justvitamins.co.uk

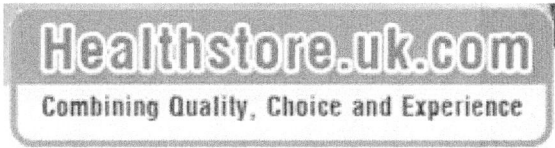

healthstore.uk.com

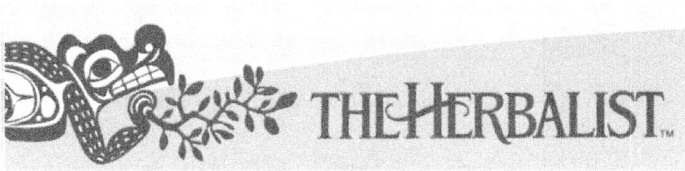

theherbalist.com

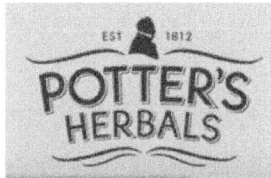

pottersherbals.co.uk

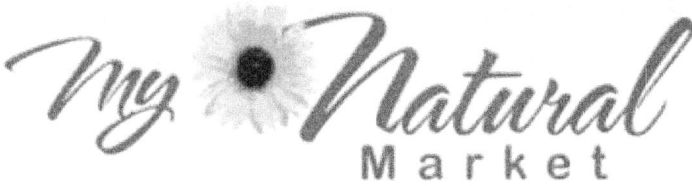

mynaturalmarket.com

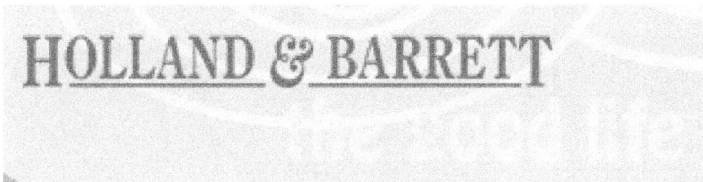

hollandandbarrett.com

FAQ

1. Which is the best medical option for treating chronic hepatitis B?

According sources (e.g. <u>hepb.org/patients/hepatitis_b_treatment.htm</u>), the following drugs are approved for hepatitis B treatment in the U.S.:

Interferon Alpha (Intron A) is given by injection several times a week for six months to a year, or sometimes longer. The drug can cause side effects such as flu-like symptoms, depression, and headaches. Approved 1991 and available for both children and adults.

Pegylated Interferon (Pegasys) is given by injection once a week usually for six months to a year. The drug can cause side effects such as flu-like symptoms and depression. Approved May 2005 and available only for adults.

Lamivudine (Epivir-HBV, Zeffix, or Heptodin) is a pill that is taken once a day, with few side effects, for at least one year or longer. Approved 1998 and available for both children and adults.

Adefovir Dipivoxil (Hepsera) is a pill taken once a day, with few side effects, for at least one year or longer. Approved September 2002 for adults. Pediatric clinical trials are in progress.

Entecavir (Baraclude) is a pill taken once a day, with few side effects, for at least one year or longer. Approved April 2005 for adults. Pediatric clinical trials are in progress.

Telbivudine (Tyzeka, Sebivo) is a pill taken once a day, with few side effects, for at least one year or longer. Approved October 2006 for adults.

Tenofovir (Viread) is a pill taken once a day, with few side effects, for at least one year or longer. Approved August 2008 for adults.

Herbal remedies that work well for chronic hepatitis B, and their symptoms, include:

- Neem

155

- Flaxseed
- Turmeric
- St. John's Wort
- Licorice Root

2. Do herbal treatments of HIV actually work?

There have been many studies into the effect of herbal treatments, in particular Black Seed, with *very* positive results. Of course, you will need to consult your doctor to ensure that none of the herbal remedies will affect your traditional medication, but as with any illness, it cannot hurt to strengthen your immune system and give your body a better chance at fighting off infection.

3. What is the best herbal treatment for throat infection?

Many herbal remedies work to fight the symptoms of influenza, in particular sore throats. The following are considered to be among the most successful:

- Honey
- Lemon
- Echinacea
- Garlic
- Zinc

4. Can you take Goldenseal without interfering with antibiotics?

It is always advisable to check with your doctor before taking any herbal remedy to ensure it doesn't interact with any medication you are taking. A study conducted by the University of Maryland (umm.edu/health/medical/altmed/herb/goldenseal), suggests that Goldenseal may affect the following:

- Cyclosporine
- Digoxin
- Tetracycline
- Anticoagulants
- Warfarin (Coumadin)
- Plavix (Clopidogrel)
- Aspirin
- Some chemotherapy drugs

- Some drugs to treat HIV
- Amitriptyline (Elavil)
- Cimetidine (Tagamet)
- Cisapride (Propulsid)
- Clarithromycin (Biaxin)
- Diltiazem (Cardizem)
- Donepezil (Aricept)
- Erythromycin
- Fexofenadine (Allegra)
- Fluoxetine (Prozac)
- Indinavir (Crixivan)
- Loperamide (Imodium)
- Lovastatin (Mevacor)
- Metoprolol (Lopressor, Toprol XL)
- Olanzapine (Zyprexa)
- Ranitidine (Zantac)
- Sildenafil (Viagra)
- Tramadol (Ultram)
- Trazodone (Desyrel)
- Triazolam (Halcion)

5. What are the best herbal antivirals to treat the herpes virus?

There are many herbal antivirals that work to fight the herpes simplex virus, but these are suggested to be the best:

- Zinc
- Lemon Balm
- Astragalus Root

6. Are there herbal remedies to get rid of warts?

Warts are caused by the *Human Papillomavirus.*

The following herbal remedies are considered the best for wart treatments:

- Apple Cider Vinegar
- Milkweed

- Banana
- Vitamin C
- Basil
- Honey
- Potato
- Pineapple

7. What is the best way to get rid of a cold naturally?

The following tips should help you get rid of a cold naturally:

- Get lots of sleep.
- Consume hot liquids.
- Blow your nose, the right way, frequently.
- Apply a saltwater gargle.
- Avoid extended travel, especially flying.
- Use an extra pillow when you sleep.
- Take hot showers.
- Use hot and cold compresses on infected sinuses.

There are also many herbal antivirals that can help with the symptoms and to fight off the virus. The "Top 45 Antiviral Herbs" chapter discusses many of these in detail.

8. What is the recommended dosage for garlic supplements?

The standard dosage is 600 mg 3 times a day, but this is dependent on your condition and other medication you're taking. Always consult your doctor when it comes to dosage for herbal remedies.

9. What are the best home remedies to detox the body?

The following list is among the most successful home detox remedies:

- Green Smoothies
- Raw Juices
- Lemon Juice
- Green Tea
- Licorice Root
- Turmeric

10. Is it okay to take herbal supplements along with antibiotics?

Many herbal supplements actually support the work of antibiotics, but it is always best to consult your doctor before combining supplements with traditional medication.

11. What are the most effective plant-based herbal antivirals?

There are many brilliantly effective plant-based herbal antivirals. The "Top 45 Antiviral Herbs" chapter of this book examines many of them in detail. According to some sources, these are suggested to be the best:

- Oil of Oregano
- Garlic
- Goldenseal
- St. John's Wort

12. How do herbal remedies fight against viruses?

Most herbal antivirals prevent the cells affected by the virus from reproducing and spreading the infection further. They work more successfully than traditional antivirals because they don't harm and kill off the infected cells. Instead, they treat them.

13. What are the best herbal antivirals to treat bronchitis?

Bronchitis is a respiratory disease affecting the bronchial passages in the lungs by causing swelling and inflammation within the mucous membranes. It is suggested that the following herbal remedies are the most successful:

- Honey
- Oregano
- Salt Water
- Ginger
- Orange Juice
- Turmeric
- Garlic
- Eucalyptus
- Onion

14. How is Covid-19 transmitted? And how did it start?

Coronavirus (Covid-19) is spread through respiratory droplets containing the virus, which are spread through person-to-person contact or through the air – when a person coughs or sneezes. When these droplets get onto the skin and somehow to the nose, mouth, or eyes of a healthy person, or they breathe these droplets, they get infected.

According to current evidence, the virus originated in Wuhan, China, in December 2019. The precise source of the virus is still unknown, but preliminary studies have linked the virus to bats that have been said to have passed it to another animal (most scientists think it is the pangolin) in one of the wet markets in Wuhan. By consuming the pangolin meat, the virus was contracted by a human, who then spread it to others.

15. Can dogs spread Covid-19 to humans?

While dogs and other pets can get coronavirus, there is no evidence supporting the notion that these animals can spread the virus to humans.

16. Do face masks protect against Covid-19? If so, which face masks are best?

Face masks protect against Covid-19, but not all face masks. The most effective face masks for respiratory illnesses like Covid-19 are certified surgical masks and N95 respirators. Other kinds of masks, such as ones that are homemade, don't demonstrate sufficient protection against this virus.

17. Are animals responsible for Covid-19 in people?

Yes. Like most other novel viruses, including MERS-COV, to which we're not immune, Covid-19 originated from animals, most likely bats, which then transmitted it to other animals, most likely the pangolin.

CONCLUSION

So as you can see from this book, herbal antivirals are a great alternative to conventional medicine when it comes to helping your body fight off viral infections. They have fewer side effects; they have a much more widespread availability; and they continually build up your immune system. These antivirals work by protecting the healthy cells from the virus, stopping it from affecting your body further. The difference from traditional antivirals is that they don't damage the infected cells.

There are many ways that you can consume these natural antivirals. Of course, there are the tablets, medicines, and oils, but there are also a lot of foods, herbs, and spices that can be incorporated into your everyday diet to ensure that you are always protected. After all, there can't be any downsides to making your body healthier and better able to fight anything that threatens it! Of course, you will need to consult your doctor to confirm that the herbal and natural remedies you seek out are suitable for you, but once you have made the lifestyle change, you won't want to go back.

ABOUT THE AUTHOR

Mary Jones became interested in herbal remedies early on in her life. After becoming frustrated with the ineffectiveness and sometimes severe side effects of synthetic remedies, she started researching whether or not natural cures could be made to the same effect, without the use of synthetic means. After dedicating years of her life to research, learning from natural remedies masters, as well as from doctors that use natural cures to help their patients, she decided it was time to share the knowledge she had gathered with the world.

One of Mary's life goals is to make the world a better, happier place, and her writings are definitely a testament to that. She does not want to keep all of her research and discoveries to herself. She has elected to share them, in a format that makes them available to just about everyone. And instead of talking about just the unknown or difficult to find herbs, as many naturalists do, she has selected remedies that anyone can make, so that every person can make themselves healthier, easily and inexpensively. Mary's books aren't just about theory; they are about practice – actually fighting infections and ailments naturally!